Harold G. Koenig, MD

Chronic Pain
Biomedical and Spiritual
Approaches

Pre-publication
REVIEWS,
COMMENTARIES,
EVALUATIONS . . .

"**K**oenig has done it again! This book expertly combines the latest scientific information with heartwarming, personal stories of people dealing with chronic pain on a daily basis. Koenig's personal experience with pain as a clinician and a patient adds depth and perspective to the discussion that you will not find in other books. The book also addresses the spiritual aspects of coping with chronic pain, including an insightful section on prayer. Essential reading for anyone with chronic pain or anyone who has loved ones with chronic pain."

Dana E. King, MD
Associate Professor of Family Medicine, Medical University of South Carolina; Author, *Faith, Spirituality, and Medicine: Toward the Making of the Healing Practitioner*

"**D**r. Koenig explores the complexities of chronic pain from a personal and from a biomedical perspective. As a physician who both treats patients with and who himself suffers from chronic pain, Dr. Koenig's personal experience and professional judgment add important insights for chronic pain sufferers. The case studies he describes illustrate how medicine has failed pain sufferers, but the information he provides suggests that a broader approach, integrating advances in pain treatment with complementary medicine and spiritual support, can provide hope and relief for people who live with pain."

Robert Friedman, MD, FACP, DABPM
Attending Physician, Cooper Pain Medicine Service, UMDNJ, Camden, NJ

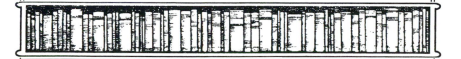

More pre-publication
REVIEWS, COMMENTARIES, EVALUATIONS . . .

"In *Chronic Pain*, Harold Koenig has written a book authoritative for his colleagues in their medical practice and supportive of chronic pain sufferers. His use of the latest research into chronic pain and his objectively organized presentation of the global character of this pain and its management earn *Chronic Pain* a place on the reference shelf of the physician.

Dr. Koenig's own experience with chronic pain helps the reader suffering from chronic pain to recognize a fellow sufferer. His description of the reach of pain into the psychological and spiritual life is one with which the reader can identify. The treatment of alternative and complementary medicine is objective. Koenig recognizes that chronic pain can deepen the understanding of a person's relationship with Christ. An appendix of numerous healing scriptures is valuable to the patient and caregiver alike."

Howard E. Mueller, MDiv, LITTD
Senior Consultant,
LCMS Health Ministries,
The Lutheran Church—Missouri Synod

"This is a very remarkable book. With the credibility that comes from high medical expertise, deep religious faith, and the experience of chronic pain, these pages present us face-to-face with a physician and a man of faith who is also a patient. I have never seen anything like it, and I have seen few books with such a capacity to bring light into darkened rooms and life into the souls of the suffering. If Harold Koenig's life experience of scholarship and service achieve nothing more, this book brings it to a focus that offers practical and reflective aid to many thousands of those for whom pain is an everyday matter. I hope they read it!"

Nigel M. de S. Cameron
Founding Editor, *Ethics and Medicine;*
Dean, The Wilberforce Forum

The Haworth Pastoral Press®
An Imprint of The Haworth Press, Inc.
New York • London • Oxford

Chronic Pain
Biomedical and Spiritual Approaches

THE HAWORTH PASTORAL PRESS
Religion and Mental Health
Harold G. Koenig, MD
Senior Editor

Chronic Pain
Biomedical and Spiritual Approaches

Harold G. Koenig, MD

To Freda –
God bless –
Hal Koenig

The Haworth Pastoral Press®
An Imprint of The Haworth Press, Inc.
New York • London • Oxford

Published by

The Haworth Pastoral Press®, an imprint of The Haworth Press, Inc., 10 Alice Street, Binghamton, NY 13904-1580.

PUBLISHER'S NOTE
Identities and circumstances of individuals discussed in this book have been changed to protect confidentiality.

All scripture quotations, unless otherwise indicated, are taken from the *HOLY BIBLE, NEW INTERNATIONAL VERSION. NIV*. Copyright 1973, 1978, 1984 by International Bible Society. Used by permission of Zondervan Publishing House. All rights reserved.

Cover design by Jennifer M. Gaska.

Library of Congress Cataloging-in-Publication Data

Koenig, Harold George.
    Chronic pain: biomedical and spiritual approaches / Harold G. Koenig.
        p. cm.
    Includes bibliographical references and index.
    ISBN 0-7890-1638-9 (alk. paper)—ISBN 0-7890-1639-7 (soft)
    1. Chronic pain. 2. Chronic pain—Psychological aspects. I. Title

RB127 .K64 2002
616'.0472—dc21

2002069061

To my wife, Charmin, my son, Jordan,
and my daughter, Rebekah,
who are my joy and love

ABOUT THE AUTHOR

Harold G. Koenig, MD, is Director and founder of the Center for the Study of Religion/Spirituality and Health at Duke University, where he is also Associate Professor of Medicine and tenured Associate Professor of Psychiatry. Dr. Koenig has published extensively in mental health, geriatrics, and religion, over 150 scientific peer-reviewed articles, 35 book chapters, and 16 books. He is editor of the *International Journal of Psychiatry in Medicine* and is founder and editor-in-chief of the monthly newspaper *Research News & Opportunities in Science and Theology.* His research on religion and health has been featured on all of the major United States television news networks, on National Public Radio, on the BBC, on the CBC, and in over 135 national/international newspapers and magazines. In September 1998, Dr. Koenig was invited to give testimony before the United States Senate concerning the health benefits of religion and spirituality. His latest books include *The Healing Power of Faith: Science Explores Medicine's Last Great Frontier; The Healing Connection; The Handbook of Religion and Health: A Century of Research Reviewed;* and *The Link Between Religion and Health: Psychoneuroimmunology and the Faith Factor.*

CONTENTS

Introduction:
What Is This Book About?

Laura sat restlessly on the edge of a black leather sofa in my office at Duke University Medical Center. She was experiencing severe pain in her right hip, a discomfort that had been with her for many months and was beginning to wear her down. She wondered why she had to go through such suffering. "What did I do to deserve this, God?" she cried out during moments of frustration, echoing the words of Job in the Bible, searching for answers that no one could give her. People at church had prayed for her, but apparently to no avail. It seemed as though her faith had failed her.

She was now seeing me, a psychiatrist, only out of desperation. She was already taking as much pain medication as her medical doctor could safely prescribe, but it hardly took the edge off the pain. Laura, a woman in her early forties with rheumatoid arthritis, was in my office because she didn't know where else to go. Her doctor had given her my phone number, saying that there was nothing more that he could do. She looked so hopeless, fidgeting to find a position that would ease her pain—the same pain that had been there when she ate lunch, when she awoke, when she went to bed the night before, and the day before that, and before that.

Laura was not the first chronic pain patient I'd seen that day. The patient before her, Bob, was a large man in his late thirties whose back was injured several years ago in a crushing spinal injury while on the job as a garbage truck supervisor. He had a wife and two children to support but could no longer work because of the pain—pain that persisted despite having undergone two complicated back surgeries and taking a handful of pain pills several times a day. He described the pain sometimes as a hot poker pressing into the bottom of his foot, and other times as having his leg in a metal vise that was slowly being screwed shut. He felt embarrassed because he could not carry out his duties as husband and father; he had tried to carry out

1

these duties—many times—but the pain stopped him. Going to church ended months ago when he could no longer sit during the services. His marriage, his friendships, and his self-esteem were all slowly disintegrating. Now, in addition to the physical pain from which he could not escape, waves of increasingly intense emotional pain threatened to engulf him.

Why is pain so distressing? Pain is distressing not only because of the physical discomfort it causes, but also because of the limitations it places on a person's daily life. The physical disability brought on by chronic pain interferes with social relationships, family life, and positive feelings about oneself. Those limitations include difficulty concentrating and performing normal physical activities, and interference with work, hobbies, and social interactions. This prevents the person from doing the things that give life meaning, purpose, and pleasure. The result, depression and hopelessness, often further interferes with activity. Consequently, a cycle of pain, depression, and decreased activity sets in, creating a downward spiral into a void of darkness.

This book is about people such as Laura and Bob, and about the treatments that are now available to help them. Meant to be both inspirational and practical, *Chronic Pain* will provide a wealth of information about the different types of pain and their causes; the effect of pain on the person's mind, body, and spirit; and the way to get control over pain, using a combination of medical, surgical, psychological, social, and spiritual strategies.

Pain can easily become a giant that intimidates and threatens to take control over every aspect of life, but this does not have to be so, even if complete pain relief is not possible. Although seeking immediate relief and total freedom from pain is preferable, most people with chronic pain must learn to live with it, cope with it, manage it, and avoid allowing their entire lives to be dominated by it. This does not mean that hope for total healing and relief should be discarded. Instead, understand that no false promises of cure are offered in this book, but rather practical, up-to-date medical, psychological, and spiritual information is shared to help people deal with pain better— even if it doesn't go away.

As a seasoned physician, I have a healthy skepticism for the value of medication and any treatment that interferes with the body's natural healing processes. The human body is finely balanced and tuned to deal with disease and aberrations. Anything that upsets this fragile balance can create problems—I've seen it many times. People with chronic pain are often placed on medications at inappropriate doses that are either too high or too low, undergo surgical procedures that are wrong for their particular condition, or spend thousands of dollars on alternative medicines that promise relief. Many continue to experience pain, but now also suffer from the additional burden of medical or surgical side effects.

Nevertheless, there is an important place for medication, for psychological and behavioral treatments, and sometimes for carefully selected surgical procedures, but they must be the right ones for the particular pain condition that is present. Also, a wide array of new scientific advances is just on the horizon that will revolutionize the treatment of pain in the future. Health professionals, religious professionals, and chronic pain sufferers themselves need to be aware of these advances in pharmacology, behavioral treatments, and surgery, because it will open up a whole new world of possible treatments.

Furthermore, misconceptions (partial truths) about pain management abound, especially among those with strong religious backgrounds. Four of these misconceptions follow: (1) do not take pain medication (or don't take enough of it) for fear of becoming addicted; (2) pain should be dealt with only in spiritual terms, and taking medication for pain relief is relying on something other than God; (3) pain should not be relieved because it results in spiritual growth; and (4) if you still have pain, then your faith is not strong enough.

Such ideas are held with the best intentions: people trying to be faithful to their understanding of religious doctrines. Nevertheless, they underestimate the complexity of spiritual, psychological, and biological factors, each of which plays a prominent role in chronic pain.

This book reviews the treatments available for pain, including prescription and nonprescription pain medication; herbal treatments, vitamins, and other botanicals; therapeutic touch, acupuncture, use of magnets, and other alternative treatments; surgical and related procedures; and new technologies enabling people with chronic pain to adapt to work and family roles more effectively. No text previously has attempted to address comprehensively the biomedical, psychological, behavioral, and spiritual dimensions of pain. However, the neglect of any one of these aspects ultimately leads to problems in all four areas. Successful pain control also requires self-discipline and a balanced schedule of activity and rest. This book will provide information to help relieve pain, emotionally cope with pain, behaviorally adapt to pain, and spiritually grow from pain.

WHO SHOULD READ THIS BOOK?

This book was written to speak to a broad audience of professionals and *especially* to people living with chronic pain and the families of those pain sufferers. It will be useful for health care professionals (physicians, nurses, social workers, and health educators) and religious professionals (chaplains, pastors, and other religious caregivers) who serve on the front line helping those in chronic pain. The comprehensive manner in which the topic is examined and the specific pharmacological, psychosocial, surgical, and spiritual strategies for managing pain provide a wealth of information and insight for these professionals.

This book will have special relevance for people who themselves battle with chronic pain. Information is provided here that will help them speak intelligently with doctors about the management of their pain. In today's health care environment, the ten-minute office visit has become the norm (often after having to wait for several months to get an appointment and several hours in the waiting room before the appointment). During such brief encounters, little time is available for questions and explanations. Many physicians do not have special expertise or training in this area and may not be aware of the newest information about medical and surgical treatments for pain. Therefore people in chronic pain need to be proactive, learning what they can about the causes of their pain and available treatments, and then presenting these findings to their physicians. The more specific and direct questions are, the greater the likelihood that doctors can help.

This text will likewise be an invaluable resource to family members who need to be better informed about the nature, causes, and treatment of chronic pain to be more effective advocates for their loved ones. Furthermore, insight into the nature of chronic pain will facilitate compassion and understanding, which will enable family members to be more supportive and to help them feel better about themselves as well.

Although pain is not a very attractive topic (the kind of subject read for fun), it is extremely common and deeply rooted in the real world in which we live. Pain is an experience we would never take on voluntarily, yet it has the potential to help us achieve incredible personal growth. It also has the potential to destroy. This is an intense war in which there are real winners and real losers. The people who lose are those who allow pain to dominate them, wear them down, and drive them to self-destruction. The people who win are those who won't give up, who find purpose and meaning in their pain, who use the pain to deepen and mold their character to make them more sensitive, more compassionate, and more deeply spiritual.

MY STORY

I am both a registered nurse and a physician with special training in the treatment of physical problems of older adults, especially those who suffer from chronic pain and disability. I am also a psychiatrist trained to help older adults overcome the emotional problems that often accompany pain, disability, and other losses associated with aging. In addition, I am a research scientist who for many years has studied the diagnosis, course, and treatment of depression in persons with painful, crippling medical illnesses. Over the past fifteen years I have taken a special interest in studying the effects of religious faith and prayer on the emotional health of those with physical problems. Thus, my medical training, clinical experience, and research interests through the years all have focused on helping people understand and overcome emotional and physical pain.

Finally, I myself suffer with chronic pain and disability resulting from a relatively rare rheumatic condition that I developed in my early thirties. I've received the best medical attention available anywhere in the world. Many, many people have recommended to me an assortment of "curative" treatments, healing potions, and spiritual strategies for relief. Unless one has struggled with the discomfort, disability, and fear of chronic pain, it is difficult to really understand what an enormous impact it has on life.

I was born into a family that emphasized hard physical work. But I learned to enjoy working and soon utilized my above-average physical abilities in high school by joining the wrestling and football teams. When I went on to college, I continued physical endurance training by lifting weights, swimming, and boxing (including a brief bout with a former featherweight U.S. boxing champion). Throughout my young adulthood I would exercise regularly, sometimes swimming a mile a day either in local swimming pools or in irrigation canals (sometimes even in the middle of winter). My educational training took me to Africa, where I hiked up and down the mountainous bush country of Tanzania conducting research on tropical butterflies, and later even scaled the 19,000-foot peak of Mount Kilimanjaro. Physical activity was my life and my life was physical activity—not a day would pass that I did not engage in some form of vigorous exercise.

In my late teens, as a result of wrestling and football, I developed a painful inflammation in the water sacs that surrounded my right knee (called bursitis). This persisted on and off throughout my twenties, and during my early thirties I started developing tendinitis in my ankles, requiring that I tape them for support when walking. Despite this, I continued exercising, playing tennis, swimming, and mountain climbing, scaling a 14,000-foot peak in Colorado. Slowly, the tendinitis spread to my wrists and then shoulders and back, gradually restricting more and more of my activity.

I didn't really begin to experience much pain, however, until my mid- to late forties when I began to have muscle spasms in my back and neck. By then it had become obvious that the local flares of bursitis and tendinitis reflected a more general condition that was eventually diagnosed as a rheumatoid condition related to psoriasis. At the age of forty-seven, I developed a severe myositis of my upper left arm associated with excruciating pain. Unlike many of my patients, however, I did have periods of relief from pain—particularly when my mind was focused on work. At night, though, the pain would intermittently return, requiring the placement of ice packs on my upper arms or a vibrating heating pad on my back (in addition to the anti-inflammatory medications I had taken for years).

As the pain began to disrupt my ability to move about independently (with flare-ups in my ankles, hips, and shoulders), it began to have more and more of an impact on my work and family life. I coped pretty well with the wrist tendinitis by obtaining voice-activated software for my computer that enabled me to write papers and letters without typing. This did not help, however, when I needed to see patients in the hospital, go to departmental meetings, supervise my research assistants, or give lectures in the hospital or in distant cities. So I bought a transport chair (a collapsible wheelchair with small wheels) and carried it in my car, asking for help from others to push me wherever I needed to go. Sometimes they were glad to provide assistance; other times they were irritated and obviously burdened by my requests. Being pushed in the hospital or through airports in my chair, I couldn't help but feel as though people were looking at me— perhaps it was more my own imagination and self-consciousness, perhaps overinterpreting stray glances and natural curiosity. Nevertheless, I felt humiliated.

Things were no better at home. My young wife had to take on extra responsibilities around the house and yard that she had not planned on when we got married. I could see the strain it was creating on her, which she handled better sometimes than others. I was also besieged by requests from my five-year-old daughter and eleven-year-old son to play with them—which I desperately wanted to do, and sometimes did anyway, paying for it later.

"Please, play soccer with me, Daddy!" My daughter would beg.

"Let's wrestle, Dad," was my son's incessant plea. Sometimes I would wrestle with him using my one good limb (the left leg that was not as affected as the right); unfortunately, other limbs would often get involved during these skirmishes. Consequently, I had to cut down on that activity. I even had difficulty playing computer games with my kids because the repeated finger and hand movements would cause flare-ups of wrist pain.

Friendships were also difficult to maintain, and any social setting was a strain—because I was different. Because my ankles would quickly inflame with use, I could not stand up for more than a couple of minutes. I had to walk rapidly into church or other social settings and sit down quickly to get the pressure off my ankles. Others would stand and talk, but I had to sit. Offers of handshakes were commonly avoided when my wrists were sore or when I was fearful that too vigorous or sincere a greeting might traumatize them. This reinforced my natural tendency toward introversion and quickly led to social isolation. I avoided going out because I couldn't do things other people did. I looked at others who could walk freely without assistance or pain, and I envied them. All of this will sound hauntingly familiar to anyone with chronic pain.

I've learned a lot on my own personal journey and in my medical practice caring for others with chronic pain and disability. Without a doubt, my religious faith has been and continues to be the foundation that keeps me going and shelters me from despair. In the pages ahead I will share with you what I've learned about the causes and treatments for chronic pain. I will suggest how to cope with the pain emotionally and to compensate for it in different ways. More than that, and perhaps most important, I will share what I've learned spiritually on this journey—the journey that I would never in a million years have chosen to take, but the one that has made me who I am.

Chapter 1

Pain Is a Common Problem

As I struggle with pain in my own world, I frequently forget how many others also suffer from this problem—many with much worse symptoms and more constant pain than I have. Those of us who have pain are indeed not alone. A recent survey by the American Pain Society found that approximately 10 percent of Americans experience moderate to severe non–cancer-related chronic pain,[1] a figure that may reach 20 percent if milder forms of chronic pain and cancer-related pain are included (nearly 50 million people, half of whom have suffered for more than five years).[2] Studies show that chronic pain is a major health care and social problem[3] and is perhaps the most common reason that people see doctors. Nearly 90 percent of all persons over age forty show beginning signs of arthritis or rheumatism, and 70 percent of persons over age sixty-five have X-ray evidence of osteoarthritis.[4]

Furthermore, the number of elderly people in the United States and around the world is rising rapidly. In 1999, according to a recent United Nation's report, there were approximately 45 million persons aged sixty or older in the United States and nearly 600 million worldwide. By 2040 to 2050, those numbers will increase to nearly 100 million in the United States and 2 billion worldwide. In some areas of Europe, over 40 percent of the population will be over age sixty by that time (Italy, Spain, Czechoslovakia, Romania, and others).[5] This means millions and millions of people in my generation (baby boomers born between 1945 in 1967) and in the generation before mine (born between World War I and World War II) either suffer or will suffer from long-term pain of some kind. Chronic pain is becoming a huge international problem.

PAIN COMPLAINTS IN THE COMMUNITY

Studies have examined the frequency of pain complaints in the general population and the kinds of conditions that cause pain. In 1993, a study of 13,538 randomly selected persons of all ages living in the United States found that the top three physical symptoms (excluding those related to the menstrual cycle) were joint pain (36.7 percent), back pain (31.5 percent), and headache (24.9 percent).[6] Of the pain symptoms reported, 84 percent either interfered with daily living, prompted the taking of medication, or forced the person to see a physician. Physical causes for the pain could not be identified for nearly one-third of symptoms. Other studies indicate that nearly 80 percent of Americans will experience low back pain at some point in their lives and in 30 percent that pain will be chronic, making it the third leading cause of disability for those of employment age.[7]

Pain is also common in populations outside of the United States. A recent World Health Organization survey of 26,000 medical outpatients from around the world found that 22 percent indicated they had experienced several months of pain during the previous year. More than 25 percent of patients attending primary care centers in Germany, Brazil, Turkey, France, and the Netherlands reported that pain was present most of the time for a period of six months or longer during the previous year.[8] In Santiago, Chile, no fewer than 33 percent of patients reported chronic pain (41 percent of women patients).

Many, then, suffer from conditions that cause chronic pain. These people frequently go from doctor to doctor, desperate to find relief. In fact, some experts believe that the increase in the popularity of complementary or alternative medicine in this country is primarily due to these people seeking help outside of the traditional health care system. Despite the hundreds of thousands who swear they have been helped, little scientific evidence shows that alternative or nontraditional methods of pain relief have *persistent* benefit.[9]

PAIN IN THE YOUNG AND OLD

Studies have shown that no significant differences exist between the way that young and older people perceive pain. However, when studies compare younger and older subjects with similar kinds of conditions, older persons are less likely to complain about pain.[10] This is true for a number of reasons. Impaired memory, decreased concentration, depression, difficulty hearing, and other problems with communication interfere with the reporting of pain.[11] Underreporting of pain may also be a problem in older adults belonging to minority groups (African Americans, Hispanics, etc.) because of differences in emotional expression or language. Members of these groups may also lack knowledge about pain treatment and sometimes have excessive fears regarding addiction to pain medication. The conditions that cause pain are a lot more common in later life, when 25 to 80 percent of people experience pain symptoms (depending on setting).[12] The most likely causes of chronic pain in older adults are arthritis, bone and joint disorders, back problems, and other chronic health conditions.

Pain is especially common among people who live in nursing homes, where between 45 percent and 80 percent of residents report substantial pain that is not adequately treated.[13] In fact, 34 percent of these patients indicate that they are in *constant* pain.[14] In a review of fourteen studies concerning the treatment of pain in nursing homes, pain was present in 49 percent to 83 percent of residents.[15] Reports of pain increase as people approach death. About two-thirds of all people have pain in their last month of life (compared to about 25 percent of people in the general population).[16] According to several studies, pain reaches its greatest intensity approximately two days before death.[17]

USE OF PAIN MEDICINE

Roughly 20 percent (one in five) of persons aged sixty-five or older take painkillers (called analgesics) several times per week.[18] Almost two-thirds (65 percent) of those 7.5 million seniors have taken analgesics for more than six months. Almost half (45 percent) of those taking pain medicine have seen three or more doctors for help with their pain in the past five years.[19] Among seniors who take medication for chronic pain, seven of ten take over-the-counter (OTC) drugs, the most common of which is acetaminophen (Tylenol) followed by nonsteroidal anti-inflammatory drugs (NSAIDs) and aspirin. Although many also take prescription drugs, more than one in four experience side effects from those drugs. It is not surprising, then, that when a new pain-relieving arthritis drug such as Celebrex (celecoxib) or Vioxx (rofecoxib) is approved for general use, it becomes the best-selling drug in America within six months. Treatment of pain has become a huge pharmaceutical industry.

There is much room for optimism, however, as safer and more effective drug treatments for pain are being marketed by pharmaceutical companies almost every year. Studies suggest that even among cancer patients, appropriate use of the World Health Organization's treatment protocol can provide pain relief for 90 percent using relatively simple drug therapies[20] (see Chapter 13). Despite this, many people with cancer—both on general medical/surgical wards and oncology wards—continue to suffer with pain.[21] This may be especially true for older patients with cancer who often receive their postacute care and rehabilitation in nursing homes, where the quality of care may be the poorest of any place in the health care system.[22]

Among older nursing home patients with cancer, a significant percentage has daily pain and unfortunately receives no pain medicine. In a study that examined the treatment of pain in nearly 14,000 elderly cancer patients admitted to nursing homes in the United States between 1992 and 1995, approximately 30 percent reported daily pain—including 38 percent of the young elderly (aged sixty-five to seventy-four) and 24 percent of the old elderly (aged eighty-five or over). More than one-quarter of these patients received no pain relievers. Patients over age eighty-five, African Americans, persons with memory or concentration difficulties, and those receiving multiple other medications were at greatest risk for receiving no treatment for their cancer pain. Although pain-relieving medication is taken by 27 percent to 44 percent of nursing home residents, it is evident that many more do not receive adequate treatment.

Thankfully, pain is receiving more and more attention in our health care system, according to an Associated Press report on December 26, 2000. The Joint Commission on Accreditation of Healthcare Organizations (JCAHO), which accredits acute-care hospitals, nursing homes, and even some outpatient clinics, has adopted new standards concerning the diagnosis and treatment of pain that all health care facilities have had to comply with since January 1, 2001. JCAHO wants to ensure that people have their pain assessed and managed in a state-of-the-art manner. If a health care institution fails to meet those standards, it may lose its license to operate. This move has finally given patients and family members some ammunition against an unconcerned health care system in their battle against pain. In fact, a jury recently awarded $1.5 million to the family of an eighty-five-year-old man dying of lung cancer because his doctor did not prescribe adequate pain medication during his final days.[23]

DEFINITION AND CAUSES OF PAIN

According to the International Association for the Study of Pain (IASP),[24] *pain* is the unpleasant physical sensation or emotional experience that is associated with either actual or possible damage to body tissues or nerves. This definition emphasizes both the physical and psychological components of pain. Deeply embedded in the skin, muscles, and internal organs are tiny receptors (called nociceptors) that are sensitive to heat and cold, pressure, and anything that causes damage to these tissues (cuts, pricks, blunt trauma, or rapidly growing cancerous tumors that crowd out or destroy normal cells and organs). From these tiny receptors come nerve fibers that transmit this information to the spinal cord and eventually to the brain.

Nerve fibers are divided into A-delta fibers and C-type fibers. A-delta fibers transmit information rapidly and are responsible for acute or sudden pain sensations. C-type fibers transmit sensory information more slowly and are responsible for more chronic types of pain. Once they reach the spinal cord, the pain impulses are modified and then transmitted to the brain. The brain interprets these signals to determine the severity and location of the pain. Interestingly, the brain also sends nerve fibers down the spinal cord to the cell bodies of the nerves from which the pain originated and in this way has the potential to either increase or decrease the intensity of the pain. Nerve fibers traveling down the spinal cord from the brain can release a substance called enkephalin, which prevents pain signals that come from the legs and arms from ever reaching the brain and awareness.

When a person presents with a complaint of pain to their physician, evaluation usually consists of a physical examination and laboratory tests to determine the underlying cause of the pain (see Chapter 8). Even though a true physical cause for the pain exists, in many cases the physician may not detect it. There are many reasons for this.

The doctor may lack the skill and training to diagnose the problem. Alternatively, medical science may not have evolved sufficiently to provide the physician with the adequate tools to diagnose the cause. It may simply be too early in the course of the disease for it to be recognized. If the doctor finds no physical or biological cause for the pain, then it is usually attributed to psychological factors. Consequently, pain is often categorized by physicians as either due to physical causes or to psychological problems.

Most current research indicates that pain cannot be so neatly classified into these two groups.[25] Although sudden or acute pain usually has an identifiable physical cause, the severity of chronic pain is seldom equal in intensity to the extent of tissue damage present. Some causes are simply unknown, such as certain types of chronic back pain or recurrent headache. It is indeed strange that careful physical and X-ray examination of persons with *no* pain nevertheless reveals underlying tissue damage in 30 percent of such individuals, whereas no structural damage is found in many persons with severe pain.[26]

According to some anesthesiologists (pain specialists), objectively verifiable tissue damage is not required for a report of pain to be real, and therefore there is no need for a direct linear relationship between reports of pain and physical findings.[27] Therefore, the primary role of the chronic pain specialist is as physician-educator, not as expert in performing technical procedures or administering pills. This does not mean that medication or surgical procedures such as nerve blocks play no role in pain management, but only that they should be performed as part of a comprehensive pain treatment program. The fundamental intervention of the pain specialist, then, is effective communication with language, not nerve blocks or medication. In fact, these pain specialists suggest that beliefs, expectations, and quality of interaction between patient and doctor are more important than specific medical or surgical techniques. For that reason doctors who care for people with chronic pain should receive special training in doctor/patient communication.[28] Unfortunately, few ever do.

For many conditions associated with chronic pain (i.e., pain lasting three months or longer, according to IASP), relatively little is known about the underlying biological or physical mechanisms responsible for the pain. Long-term, unrelenting pain can often result from changes in the nervous system that occur in response to earlier tissue damage.

These changes may continue to send pain impulses to the brain even after complete healing of tissue has taken place. Changes in the processing of pain signals within the nervous system may cause a person to experience severe pain in the absence of a physical cause (or in the absence of ongoing tissue destruction). Attempts to relieve the pain in such circumstances through surgical methods directed at the painful body part often fail to bring relief. Nevertheless, chronic pain may result from a number of identifiable biological, anatomic, or physiologic causes. Knowing that the pain may have a physical cause is very important for chronic pain patients because it helps combat the humiliating notion that the pain is "all in their head" or somehow due to defects in these individuals.

TYPES OF PAIN

In general, there are three basic types of pain. None of these are completely independent or separate from the other two.

Physiologic Pain

Physiologic pain (pain resulting from physical causes) results from inflammation around nerves, injury to nerves, or physical irritation of nerves. This kind of pain, whose origins can be directly linked to physical causes, is called *nociceptive* pain (from the Latin verb *nocere* which means "to injure"). Injury or damage can occur anywhere along nerve pathways—from nerve endings in the skin, to nerve roots as they enter into the spinal cord, to nerve cell bodies in the spinal cord, to nerve tracts in the spinal cord, to nerve cells in the brain, to the actual network of brain cells that enable pain to be perceived.

Physiologic pain is further divided into somatic (external body) and visceral (internal body) types of pain. Somatic pain results when nerve receptors in the skin, muscles, and deep tissues such as bone are stimulated. Usually, somatic pain is described as well localized, stabbing, aching, or gnawing. Visceral pain, on the other hand, often results from infiltration, compression, distension, or stretching of organs such as the liver, stomach, or intestines, and is often described as poorly localized, deep, squeezing, colicky, or pressurelike. The latter type of pain may be associated with nausea, vomiting, or sweating.

Neuropathic Pain

Pain can also be caused by nonnociceptive sources. This type of physiologic pain, called *neuropathic* pain, continues to cause discomfort despite a lack of ongoing tissue damage or injury. Neuropathic pain has its source within the nervous system itself and results from abnormal processing of pain signals in the spinal cord and brain. Because the pain results from abnormal nervous system processing and has no clear ongoing injury or tissue damage associated with it, neuropathic pain is extremely difficult to verify on objective testing.

This type of pain, often found in persons with chronic pain, is severe and constant, often described as a dull ache or vicelike pressure that is accompanied by paroxysms of burning pain or electric shocks. The autonomic nervous system (sympathetic and parasympathetic nerves), known to be strongly influenced by emotional state, plays an important role in this kind of pain. Examples include phantom limb pain (following limb amputation), reflex sympathetic dystrophy (resulting from immobilization of a body part to avoid pain), and a variety of postsurgical pain syndromes (following back or neck operations, joint replacement, or certain pelvic surgeries). This is the most difficult kind of pain to diagnose and treat effectively, often failing to improve even when narcotic pain relievers are taken, anesthetic nerve blocks are given, or even neurosurgical procedures performed.

Psychogenic Pain

This type of pain, in its purest form, has no physical or biological cause. It is entirely due to psychological factors and represents a way of coping with emotional distress over a life problem. The person is not conscious of the psychological nature of the pain and does not fabricate the symptom. The pain experienced by this person seems as real to him or her as that experienced by a person with true physical pain. If a person is intentionally and consciously feigning a pain symptom, this is called *malingering*. Malingering is relatively easy for pain specialists to identify and separate from other types of pain.

Neuropathic and psychogenic pain, however, are very difficult to distinguish from one another because the symptoms are almost identical and are based entirely on nonverifiable personal reports.

Atypical types of facial pain, certain kinds of low back pain, and other musculoskeletal complaints that are due to psychological stress or conflict are examples of psychogenic pain. Pain can be the result of a conversion disorder, in which a psychological conflict is expressed as a physical symptom. Again, these pain complaints are not conscious. Psychogenic pain can also result from depression (called "masked" depression), hysterical syndromes, or even from delusional beliefs (i.e., mental illness).

Combined Pain Syndromes

Most of the time, especially in those experiencing chronic pain, there is a mixture of different types of pain. For any degree of objectively verifiable physical pain, there is almost always a psychological component that influences its perception. As previously noted, the meaning of pain can either magnify or diminish the intensity of the pain.

On one hand, the pain of childbirth is often minimized because the mother is anticipating the arrival of her baby. On the other hand, the pain of arthritis or cancer may be exaggerated or magnified because it symbolizes a threat to one's future way of life or life itself. Chronic pain that is present day in and day out, that disrupts sleep, family life, and self-image, will only naturally be followed by psychological problems such as depression or anxiety. These emotional states tend to worsen the intensity of the pain, which worsens the psychological consequences, and so on, sending the sufferer into a downward spiral. Examples of combined pain syndromes include headache, fibromyalgia, and certain types of low back pain.

INFLUENCE OF THE MIND

From the previous discussion we know that the brain itself can influence the perception of pain. For at least twenty years, scientists have known that pain pathways in the spinal cord receive messages from the brain. Depending on the person's circumstances and past experiences, these inputs modulate or control the amount of pain allowed into consciousness. The intensity of pain is greatly influenced by the level of attention given to the pain (which is based on how important the person perceives the pain to be). Therefore, it is easy to understand that for any given level of objective physical pain there will be a wide range of reports of severity by different people. These subjective reports depend on setting, culture, personality, expectations, social factors, mood state, and feelings of control, as well as on the actual amount of disease or objective tissue injury.[29] Some of the factors that influence the pain experience are discussed next.

Setting of the pain. If a person experiences a wound during a fight or athletic event, he or she may hardly notice it until afterward. The person's attention is focused on survival and overcoming the opponent, and is therefore directed away from the pain. However, if a physical injury occurs within a safe setting (e.g., in the presence of family) in which nurturance is likely forthcoming, such a wound will receive great attention and be experienced as causing much discomfort.

Cultural factors. Cultural factors have long been known to influence both the perception and expression of pain. A person from a Mediterranean background may tend to complain loudly over his or her wounds, whereas a person of Irish or English descent may tolerate pain stoically, saying little about it.[30]

Personality factors. Temperament, due in part to genetic background and in part to early environmental influences, often plays an important role in the experience and expression of pain. For example, the phlegmatic individual might report pain only if it is relatively severe and disruptive, whereas the choleric individual may report the slightest discomfort as distressing and worthy of others' attention.

Expectations. People who expect to have pain often experience more of it. This is again likely due to the greater attention paid to the pain stimulus, which is then magnified in severity. Anticipation of pain may also increase muscle tension, which further enhances the pain. This works in the opposite direction for people who expect not to have pain. The mind is diverted to other things, which tends to block the perception of pain. Only when pain becomes severe does it force attention to itself. Expectations of pain have a lot to do with past experiences and with an individual's personality.

Social factors. As previously noted, pain is often magnified in settings conducive to nurturance and minimized in settings that are not. Settings conducive to nurturance include those in which people are surrounded by maternal figures. Settings that are not conducive to nurturance include gatherings of men (such as in prison or in the military) where the expression of pain is viewed as a weakness and is therefore discouraged.

Mood state. Depression is well known to increase the severity of pain because it draws attention to negative experiences and reinforces negative thinking. Hopelessness and helplessness can easily transform even moderate pain into agonizing, unbearable suffering.

Feelings of control. It is extremely important for those with chronic pain to have some sense of control over the pain. This influences the tolerability of pain. Simply having pain medicine in one's possession can relieve anxiety and decrease the need to take the medicine. If control over the pain is lost, however, a sense of desperation ensues, which only worsens both physical and emotional suffering.

Disease/objective tissue injury. Amount of tissue injury and nerve ending stimulation are powerful predictors of pain severity. People who have burned a significant portion of their skin experience severe pain since many damaged nerve receptors are sending messages of discomfort to the brain.

Thus, many factors interact with each other to determine a person's experience of pain. Because each of these factors differs in every pain patient, the primary sources of pain often become hopelessly lost or extremely difficult to identify.

PHYSICAL CAUSES OF PAIN

The most common causes of chronic pain are musculoskeletal disorders, such as ligament sprains, muscle strains, injuries to the back, and arthritis. Of the 7 million seniors who take pain medications, nearly three-quarters take them for pain from arthritis or other bone and joint problems. The second most common cause of chronic pain in persons of all ages is nerve-related or neurogenic pain. These two categories (arthritis and neurogenic pain) cover 80 to 90 percent of all chronic pain conditions experienced by Americans. Specific physical sources of pain differ depending on the age of the individual. Examples of the most common causes of pain in young, middle-aged, and older adults follow.

The most common pain complaints in younger persons involve low back discomfort, abdominal pain due to irritable bowel syndrome or spastic colitis, headache, tendinitis due to overuse syndromes, fibromyalgia, and musculoskeletal problems related to physical injuries or accidents. Less common causes of pain in younger adults are sickle-cell anemia (in African Americans), inflammatory arthritis (typically due to autoimmune disorders), multiple sclerosis, and other conditions causing irritation to nerves or nerve roots.

By middle age, arthritis-related pain becomes more common, as does pain from chronic musculoskeletal disorders. Rheumatoid arthritis and other autoimmune inflammatory disorders peak in persons aged forty to sixty years, and are especially common in women. Other causes include cancer-related pain, diabetic neuropathy (inflamed nerves due to diabetes), abdominal pain due to gastritis or peptic ulcers, and pain syndromes seen in younger adults that occur with greater frequency in middle age.

Among older adults, physical damage or objective pathology is the most common cause of pain, and psychogenic pain is more rare than in younger persons. The most frequent cause of pain is osteoarthritis of the shoulder, hip, knee, and hand joints. Recall that 70 percent of persons over sixty-five years of age have X-ray evidence of osteoarthritis and 44 percent experience pain related to it.[31] Other chronic pain syndromes in older adults result from herpes zoster infection, neuralgias (trigeminal neuralgia, occipital neuralgia), cluster headaches, temporal arteritis, rheumatoid disorders, peripheral neuropathy, peripheral vascular disease, irritable bowel, and chronic constipation. Cancer-related pain is the most feared type of pain in older adults and increases in frequency with age.

SPECIFIC PAIN SYNDROMES

The five most common syndromes that produce over 90 percent of all chronic pain are arthritis, fibromyalgia, headache, low back problems, and cancer. These conditions are briefly introduced here, and in Chapter 13 detailed information on management is provided.

Arthritis

It is important to distinguish the various kinds of arthritis, as treatments differ depending on type. The most common type of arthritis, seen more often in older persons, is *osteoarthritis*. Osteoarthritis results from the wear and tear on joints caused by many years of use. This is typically a noninflammatory arthritis characterized by progressive deterioration of cartilage that lines the contact surfaces of bones in the fingers and toes, hands and feet, wrists and ankles, elbows and knees, shoulders, hips, and spine. Factors that bring on osteoarthritis include advanced age, obesity, overuse or abuse of joints during work or sports activity, and physical trauma from accidents. For example, a runner, after many years, may develop osteoarthritis of the ankles, knees, or hips. Osteoarthritis of the spine is very common in advanced age after years of bending or stooping. Of course, the likelihood of developing osteoarthritis is also influenced by genetic factors or heredity. Osteoarthritis is often associated with joint stiffness and inactivity; treatment involves heat, exercise, regular use of involved joints, and judicious use of pain relievers.

The second kind of arthritis is due to inflammation, not wear and tear, and is more often seen in younger persons. This type of arthritis is very different from osteoarthritis both in its cause and treatment. *Inflammatory arthritis* such as rheumatoid arthritis, arthritis related to lupus erythematosis, or arthritis related to psoriasis (as in my condition), results from an autoimmune process in which the body's own immune system attacks the tendons and membranes surrounding the joint spaces. Instead of improving pain symptoms, too vigorous exercise often induces inflammation, causing further deterioration of joints and increasing pain. Careful attention to balancing activity and rest to avoid joint trauma or overuse is essential. Anti-inflammatory drugs (such as ibuprofen), steroids, and sometimes antineoplastic drugs (methotrexate), along with pain relievers such as acetaminophen, are used to help control disease activity and symptoms.

Fibromyalgia

Fibromyalgia (also called myofascial pain syndrome, fibromyositis, or fibromyitis) is a chronic musculoskeletal condition associated with pain in the muscles, tendons, and ligaments that surround joints or bone. According to the 1990 American College of Rheumatology criteria,[32] this diagnosis requires a history of widespread pain and tenderness to palpation or pressure (trigger points) in at least eleven of eighteen muscle sites for at least three months. Pain must be present both on the left and right sides of the body, above and below the waist. Pushing down with a single finger (at a force of approximately nine pounds) must elicit pain (not tenderness) at trigger points located on the backside of the head, the lower cervical spine, the upper back, around the scapula, where the ribs connect to the breastplate, around the elbows, in the upper outer quadrant of the buttocks, the hips, or the knees. This condition can be associated with fatigue, depression, and fever, when it is sometimes called chronic fatigue syndrome.

Headache

The most common form of head pain is the *tension headache*. This kind of headache is a steady ache on both sides of the head. The pain is slight to moderate in intensity, and may last hours, weeks, or months. The muscles of the head and neck are sensitive to psychological and social stress, often going into partial or full spasm during times of distress. Muscle tension causes a reduction in blood flow to the muscles. This reduced blood flow causes muscle ischemia (lack of oxygen in the tissues), resulting in the release of inflammatory substances that stimulate pain receptors. Muscle relaxants, application of hot or cold compresses, reduction of stress, and pain relievers help to reduce muscle spasms and ease discomfort.

Another common form of head pain is called a *migraine* (or vascular headache). This headache is throbbing, occurs on one side of the head, is moderate to severe in intensity, and typically lasts from four hours to three days. Migraines are thought to result from constriction of small vessels that supply blood to the brain and the membranes that cover the brain. Vascular constriction again causes ischemia or lack of oxygenation, resulting in the release of inflammatory substances that cause excessive dilation of blood vessels. The swollen blood vessels stretch and stimulate nerves located around the blood vessels, sending pain signals to the brain. Darkness, quietness, and rest may help to ameliorate the pain. Application of cold packs, drinking caffeinated beverages, or use of drugs that constrict these dilated vessels also help to relieve symptoms. There is often a genetic or hereditary component to migraines in those so predisposed, and a variety of stimuli can set off the headache—including bright lights, certain sounds and smells, alcoholic beverages, chocolate, or intense emotional states.

Low Back Pain

There are many causes of low back pain. The vertebral or spinal column in the center of the back is made up of short, blocklike cylindrical bones (called vertebrae) that are stacked one upon another. Because of this and the cushionlike discs that separate these bones, the vertebral column has both structure and flexibility to allow humans to stand upright and also bend down and twist and turn. The spinal cord is a complex conduit of nerves that extends up the center of the vertebral column and connects at the top to the brain inside the skull. Along its entire length, the spinal cord sends out nerves to the arms, legs, and rest of the body.

Spinal degenerative disc disease occurs when the soft gelatinous discs (shock absorbers) between the vertebrae are injured, lose strength, and rupture, putting pressure on nearby nerve roots that extend out from the spinal cord to the arms and legs.

Chronic postural imbalance causes back pain because it strains the ligaments that hold the vertebrae together in the vertebral column, placing unusual pressure on various muscles and increasing the risk of muscle injury or vertebral disc rupture.

Congenital vertebral disorders result when a person is born with abnormalities in the vertebrae that make up his or her vertebral column, interfering with the normal mechanical structure of the back. This places unusual stress on ligaments, muscles, and vertebral discs, making them prone to injury and wearing out.

Osteoporosis is a disease of the vertebral bones resulting from insufficient calcium in the bone that weakens the vertebrae and increases the risk of fracture or compression when placed under stress. Dietary lack of calcium and vitamin D, low levels of physical activity, and lack of estrogen after menopause all combine to bring on this bone disorder.

Compression fractures of the spine may result from motor vehicle accidents, falls, or injuries that occur during violent sporting events. Osteoporosis predisposes individuals to compression fractures in older adulthood.

As previously noted, osteoarthritis results from wear and tear on bones and on the cartilage or plasticlike covering on the bone where two different bones come into contact with each other. This often results in the deformation of bones due to bone resorption and deposition in response to physical stress. In osteoarthritis of the spine, the vertebrae that make up the vertebral column become deformed and often impinge on nerves coming off from the spinal cord causing pain.

Scoliosis is an inherited sideways curvature of the vertebral column that places unusual pressure on bones, muscles, and ligaments. These impinge on nerves exiting from the spinal cord. This is most frequently seen in adolescent girls and teenagers.

Spondylosis occurs when part of the vertebral column is shifted forward or backward resulting in pressure on the spinal cord. This is most often seen in older persons with osteoarthritis.

Spinal stenosis is a narrowing of space surrounding the spinal cord as it goes through the vertebral column. Again, this condition is seen more often in older persons with osteoarthritis.

Despite the many known causes of back pain, the primary cause is uncertain in more than 80 percent of people who present to their family physician for treatment with this complaint.[33] These patients are typically referred from one physician to another until they eventually arrive at a chronic pain clinic. It is not surprising, then, that for the vast majority of patients with back pain attending a chronic pain clinic, the cause of the pain is unclear and there is a great deal of psychological and social dysfunction present (either causing the pain, resulting from the pain, or both).[34] By this time, after many months of pain, depression is common, as are conflict with the legal system, family problems, substance abuse, and excessive health care use.

Cancer Pain

Many people with cancer experience pain. Cancer-related pain affects tens of millions of people around the world. Studies indicate that chronic pain is present in about 30 to 50 percent of patients with cancer who undergo treatment for a solid tumor and 70 to 90 percent of those with advanced disease.[35] Among those with all types of advanced cancer, moderate to severe pain is experienced by 51 percent, ranging from 43 percent in stomach cancer to 80 percent in gynecologic cancer (cervix, uterus, or ovaries). However, there is some disagreement among scientists on how often cancer patients report pain. Some studies suggest that only one-third of cancer patients with metastatic disease complain of pain that interferes with their way of life. Overall, most medical researchers agree that about two-thirds of cancer patients with advanced disease experience significant pain.

Three-quarters of chronic pain syndromes seen in people with cancer are due to a direct effect of the growing cancer. The rest are due to cancer treatments or disorders unrelated to the cancer or its treatment. Surprisingly, only a small percentage of people with cancer that has spread to the bone (metastasized) will experience pain. The most common site of bone metastasis is the spine. Back pain may result from vertebral metastasis, which may compress the spinal cord or compress exiting nerves that branch off the spinal cord.

Pain syndromes in cancer patients can be either acute (short term), when often due to procedures or therapies, or chronic (long term), when often due to tumor-related physical compression or destruction of organs or tumor-related neuropathic pain syndromes. Most chronic pain after the treatment of cancer is neuropathic in nature (i.e., due to damage done to nerves). Any cancer-related surgical procedure might lead to neuropathic pain. Alternatively, pain could be due to tumor recurrence, to a neuroma (nerve growth) at the amputation site, or to abnormalities in the nervous system's processing of impulses after amputation. Radiation therapy can cause fibrosis (scar tissue) that damages nerves and causes neuropathic pain weeks or even years after the treatment.

Pain in cancer patients usually includes multiple physical, psychological, social, spiritual, and existential domains. Each of these domains requires attention. *Palliative* care (care focused on relieving suffering) addresses all these issues and is especially appropriate for patients with progressive incurable illness. Such treatment typically involves a multidisciplinary approach (involving cancer specialists, anesthesiologists, nurses, psychologists, chaplains, etc.) as seen in some hospice programs and palliative care units.

SUMMARY

Chronic pain is common and can be categorized into different types. Physiologic pain results from physical or biological diseases, whereas psychogenic pain results from psychological or emotional causes. Neuropathic pain is a type of physiologic pain that occurs in the absence of ongoing tissue damage, and results from the abnormal processing of pain signals in the nervous system. Psychological and social factors can have an enormous influence on the perception of pain, as can culture, setting in which the pain occurs, personality, expectations, and mood state. Physiologic pain can have a number of different causes. These causes vary depending on a person's age, activity level, and heredity.

Chapter 2

A Giant Called Mr. Pain

I'd like to tell you a silly story about a giant named Mr. Pain who lived in a large, decaying old house in the middle of a thriving metropolis, Anytown, located in a faraway land called Eternal Existence. He was an unsightly fellow with a crooked wart-tipped nose, evil-looking bloodshot eyes, wild and stringy unkempt matted hair, and a terrible body odor. He had long powerful arms, a huge hairy chest, and enormous pillarlike legs—and he was very quick. Mr. Pain moved into this particular house because it was conveniently located near a city park. Here he had access to hundreds of people each day strolling along the sidewalk on their way to work, to the shopping mall, on the way to school, or simply coming to the park to play. Every so often, he would open his door, reach out with his long arms and snatch an unsuspecting individual as he or she passed by. On slow days, he would go out into the park or city streets searching for other victims.

After dragging his captives inside, Mr. Pain would tie them up and carry them down the cellar steps into his basement. He had trapped hundreds, perhaps thousands of people this way, housing them in a maze of tunnels and caves that extended from under his house deep below the city. Most of these unfortunates were taken completely by surprise. They struggled violently at first to get loose, but to no avail. The chains he used to attach their ankles to the cave walls were made of heavy glistening metal, and breaking free was next to impossible.

Soon after being seized, most people tried to bargain with the giant. If he would only release them, they promised to do whatever he wished. But the giant was not easily fooled. He knew they would keep none of their promises if he released them. Some, out of frustration, would yell at the giant whenever he came around—which he enjoyed immensely and would cause him to taunt them even more mercilessly. After awhile, having failed to struggle free or bargain their way out, the captives often became overwhelmed with sadness. They became much more manageable from that point on, but not nearly as much fun. If they survived much longer, the captives typically fell into a numb state of simply not caring about anything anymore.

Making matters worse, the giant loved to torture his hostages, at night in particular. When they fell asleep, if they dared, he would sneak down and poke them with sharp pins, stomp their legs or arms, pummel their sides and backs, or squeeze their heads in a vise that he carried in his inside coat pocket. Many could not fall asleep, fearing the giant's unpredictable actions. This constant harassment quickly took its toll, exhausting them. Many wished the giant would simply kill them and get it over with, and some plotted quietly and desperately to end their own lives.

Besides Mr. Pain, other giants lived in various parts of the city. They had funny names: Mrs. Drugaddiction, Mr. Sexaddiction, Mr. Workaholic, Mr. Materialism, Mrs. Foodaddiction, Mr. Lazybum, Mr. Moneylover, to name just a few. Each had secret places in their dwellings where they kept captives. These were linked to Mr. Pain's dungeons through a complex of underground tunnels. Similar to Mr. Pain, these giants did what they could to detain and imprison the citizens of Anytown, about one-quarter of whom had already succumbed to their temptations. They would entice the naive into their houses with all sorts of delights and pleasures, and once inside they too would tie them up and throw them into their basements. There these unfortunate souls remained for weeks, months, sometimes years. Some spent the remainder of their lives there.

A few of Mr. Pain's captives, over time, actually wore down the chains around their ankles by rubbing them against rough places on the floor or wall. Once free, they would desperately search through the tunnels for a way of escape. Unfortunately, they often became lost and disoriented in the maze—finding themselves face to face with the other giants—Mr. Drugaddiction, Mr. Alcoholism, or Mr. Suicide, who roamed the tunnels seeking to lure hopeful escapees by promising them freedom.

Mr. Pain anticipated that some of his captives would try to escape, find a way out, and get away. To prevent escapes and stop those who successfully got away from telling others about his evil deeds,

Mr. Pain arranged to have a special potion placed into the drinking water offered at various places in the tunnels. The disorientation and confusion caused by this potion not only helped to prevent escapes, but if anyone did get away, they would soon forget about the giant and the terrible experiences they had in his captivity. Having forgotten the experience, they would resume their lives as though nothing ever happened—and perhaps even be captured again.

Some of those who escaped were wise enough not to drink the tunnel water. When they tried to tell others about their experiences, though, they were often ridiculed. Things couldn't possibly be as bad as all that. They were accused of exaggerating their complaints or of making them up altogether. Few people took them seriously, so the escapees soon lost interest in telling others and after a few days returned to their routines. So Mr. Pain and the other giants continued their sinister activities with little resistance. As bleak as things seemed, though, there was reason for hope.

The city of Anytown was located in a vast land called Eternal Existence. This place was presided over by a good, wise king named Mr. Freedom. He was a kind and fair ruler who loved the people of Anytown very much and wanted them to live free and happy lives there. He knew that the time they spent in Anytown would be relatively short before they moved on to live elsewhere in Eternal Existence. In fact, he had a specific plan for each of the inhabitants of Anytown that would make their lives full and enable the entire community to prosper.

Not everyone, however, wanted to be led by Mr. Freedom. Many of the people had their own interests and little time to bother with him. Of course, this was their choice. Mr. Freedom knew both the people and the giants very well. In fact, he had written a book describing his plan for the people of Anytown. In that book he described how the people could avoid, endure, or escape from the many difficulties they faced that were imposed by the giants. This book became known as the Book of Life. Mr. Freedom encouraged everyone to read the Book of Life when they came to live in Anytown.

In addition to being a great king and fine author, Mr. Freedom was a very personable guy and wanted to be involved in the lives of his people as much as they would let him. Remember though that most citizens of the city, particularly when they had work, money, plenty to eat and drink, and lots of interesting hobbies to occupy their time, were too distracted to pay much mind to Mr. Freedom. Of course, being captured by a giant sometimes gave them more time to consider such matters.

At any moment, because of his position and power, Mr. Freedom could have done away with Mr. Pain and all the other giants, and released all the captives who were under their control. Yes, Mr. Freedom could have gotten rid of the giants and completely controlled the lives of the people of Anytown himself, preventing them from injuring or hurting each other, using alcohol, drugs, or food excessively, or preoccupying themselves with any of the many other pleasures that the giants offered.

Except for one thing. There were laws that Mr. Freedom had helped set up when the city of Anytown was established many years earlier. The laws ensured that the citizens and the giants (who in the beginning were peaceable and friendly) had certain rights. The first and foremost of those rights was the right to choose—to choose where to live, how to live, with whom to associate, and what to spend one's time and talents on. A number of regulations also resulted from that first and primary right. These laws were developed to ensure that one person's choice did not interfere with another person's choice. Everything usually worked very smoothly when everyone followed the rules, but most people didn't. All of the laws could have been followed if people had simply loved each other. But this seemed most difficult for almost everyone. They were far too concerned about their own immediate happiness and pleasure.

Mr. Freedom loved his people and wanted them to love him and to love each other. Why? Because he knew very well that this was the only way for them to experience full, happy, and contented lives in the city of Anytown, and to avoid the giants. Mr. Freedom often invited the people to accept his help. He sometimes talked to them directly and at other times sent them messages through others. Remember, however, that the people were completely free to either accept or reject his help. This was part of their right to choose.

Mr. Freedom also made sure that everyone knew about or had a copy of the Book of Life if they wanted it. The Book was important because it described the laws of living in the city of Anytown and the consequences of breaking those laws. Some of the people read it, but most did not. The giants in the city had long ago chosen to reject Mr. Freedom's help and advice. Instead, they did everything they could to subvert his activities and interfere with his intentions for the city. Therefore, the giants made great efforts to get rid of the Book, since they didn't want the people to discover the secrets to real freedom that it contained.

One of the laws in the Book, added after the giants turned to evil ways, advised the residents of Anytown not to go anywhere near the giants' houses, a law frequently disregarded. After all, the giants' houses on the outside seemed so welcoming and inviting (except Mr. Pain's, of course). Indeed, the insides of the giants' houses also seemed pleasant, as citizens wandered in and out of them. The giants were very sneaky, though. Only a few of the citizens each day—the vulnerable ones—would be seized. This was done very quietly so as not to disturb the other guests or arouse suspicion.

Mr. Freedom knew that the only way the people could truly obey the laws in the Book of Life was if he helped them do so—if they somehow allowed Mr. Freedom to change their minds and hearts. Mr. Freedom could only do that if they came to him by their own free will. Unfortunately, it was often only when they got into trouble with one of the giants or ran into other difficulties in life that the people would remember Mr. Freedom's offer or his Book.

Mr. Freedom realized that despite their continual efforts to disrupt his efforts, the giants also had rights. They had a right to live freely in the city of Anytown and go about the evil work that they had chosen to do. The first law in the Book had guaranteed that freedom. If citizens out of their own free will chose to go too near or inside the giants' houses, then the giants could not be stopped from capturing them. Because of these rights, Mr. Freedom could not interfere with the activity of the giants directly.

There was one thing, though, that really bothered Mr. Freedom. Sometimes the giants—especially Mr. Pain—would sneak out at night and capture people even if they were obeying most of the laws and staying clear of the giants' houses. This included many who knew and loved Mr. Freedom, people whom Mr. Freedom cared for deeply. It also included those who did not know Mr. Freedom, but who on their own were trying to obey the laws and lead a good life in the city of Anytown. Whenever any of these innocent people were captured, particularly his friends, Mr. Freedom himself would experience the very pain and suffering they were going through.

Because Mr. Pain was especially known for stepping outside his bounds to capture the innocent, many felt it was unfair and that he should not be allowed to get away with this. They maintained that such people had done nothing to warrant Mr. Pain's actions. It simply didn't make sense—why should these people have to suffer? They were good people obeying all the rules. Part of the answer to this question was contained in the Book of Life. The Book said quite clearly that any giant who overstepped his bounds would be ultimately punished for those actions—leading eventually to that giant's downfall. This was because of the Great Law that ruled the land.

According to the Great Law, both the giants and the citizens of Anytown were held accountable for their actions. This was true not only during the period they lived in the city Anytown, but also wherever they might live or venture throughout all time in the land of Eternal Existence. Therefore, both giants and people could be either compensated or punished at some future time for what they did while living in the city of Anytown. That is why the relatively brief period spent in Anytown was so crucial. Mr. Freedom knew that the decisions made at that time could ultimately affect a person's destiny wherever they lived from then on. Thus, even though Mr. Pain might seem to be getting away with his sinister actions that infringed upon the freedoms of the people of Anytown, he was sure to pay for it later. Similarly, people experiencing undeserved suffering at the hands of Mr. Pain—particularly if they carried their pain with courage— would experience a special reward after they completed their time in the city of Anytown.

There was another consequence of Mr. Pain's actions affecting the lives of his captives even during the time they were in Anytown. These activities by Mr. Pain would drive many people to get to know Mr. Freedom better and to study his Book more closely, ultimately freeing them, and if not freeing them then giving them knowledge that would greatly advance them wherever they would venture in the future after Anytown. Others, not knowing or believing what was promised in the Book, not knowing or believing about the life following Anytown, continued to insist that it was just unfair. They refused to acknowledge or accept the help offered by Mr. Freedom and chose instead to forge their own path. These poor souls didn't do very well when captured by the giants, particularly Mr. Pain, since they had no one to rely on for help except themselves. Although Mr. Freedom cared deeply about these people and had the power to bring companionship, encouragement, and hope to any person who called out to him, he could not come to the aid of those who refused to acknowledge him or to accept his help.

Many of the captives, even good friends of Mr. Freedom, got angry at him for not protecting them from the giants' seemingly unfair behaviors. This anger, which contributed to their unhappiness, sometimes prevented them from calling out to Mr. Freedom for help. This prevented him from coming to their rescue or sending others to comfort and help free them. Mr. Freedom would also make every effort to get them copies of the Book, which held the secrets to living in prison with greater peace, meaning, and purpose.

Previously, Mr. Pain had reluctantly agreed (in response to Mr. Freedom's threat to close him down entirely) to allow the distribution of a certain kind of root among the captives. If chewed on, this root would ease the physical discomfort and mental discouragement caused by Mr. Pain. Some of the captives, however, refused to use the root fearing that they might become dependent on it (and then they would have to suffer even more if they ever ran out of it). Other captives chewed on the root whenever they could get their hands on it, sometimes greedily taking more than their share, which typically got them into trouble. Others used the root more moderately. For them, it made a real difference. Mr. Freedom shared the joy over whatever relief the captives experienced from using the root. Chewing the root, however, relieved the pain only temporarily, and for some poor souls it did not even do that. So there was much physical and emotional suffering that remained—to Mr. Pain's satisfaction and to Mr. Freedom's sadness.

There was a man named Anyone who lived in the city of Anytown. He was a hardworking fellow who lived by himself and was known for his kindness to strangers. Anyone as a child had heard about the giants from his mother, and so carefully he avoided their neighborhoods. He had also heard of Mr. Freedom, but did not know him very well. His mother, however, was very close to Mr. Freedom. As a young boy, Anyone would find her talking to Mr. Freedom, something she seemed to do a lot, especially when her children were in trouble. She had great respect for Mr. Freedom, and carefully followed the laws in the Book of Life. To Anyone, these rules and regulations seemed pretty difficult to follow. His mother had told him it was easy for her because of the advice and help that Mr. Freedom gave. In fact, her close relationship with him had caused her to *want* to follow these rules.

One day, when Anyone was minding his own business walking home from work through the park, Mr. Pain sneaked up from behind a bush, grabbed him, and carted him off to his house. Tied and secured in Mr. Pain's cave, Anyone finally realized what had happened. At first he was angry, frustrated, and became discouraged, as did the other prisoners. It was not long, however, before he remembered what his mother had read to him from the Book when he was a child. So he called out to Mr. Freedom, asking him for help, since there seemed nothing else left to do. Suddenly, to his surprise, a small copy of the Book of Life appeared at his feet. When he picked it up, out fell a short letter addressed to him from Mr. Freedom. He opened it and read:

> Dear friend,
>
> Read this book carefully. You will find help in it for your present situation. Remember that just as I love your mother, I also love you. So don't ever hesitate to call on me, whether you are in trouble or not, for I want you to get to know me and to love me as I love you.

While Mr. Freedom could not directly free the prisoners taken by giants such as Mr. Pain, the giants also could not prevent Mr. Freedom from communicating with Anyone if he called out. They did, however, try to make such communication difficult. Because of the tortures he inflicted day and night, Mr. Pain made it especially hard for Anyone to talk to Mr. Freedom or read his Book. Nevertheless, Anyone persisted in calling out to Mr. Freedom in spite of his suffering. Soon, Anyone heard Mr. Freedom speaking to him in a small quiet voice, urging him to take up the Book of Life and turn to a certain page. Anyone opened the Book to the place where he was instructed and began to read:

> Should you be taken captive by a giant and thrown into a prison, strike up a conversation with the fellow next to you and get to

know him. Listen carefully to that person's life story and especially how he was captured. Encourage that person and share
with him some of the passages in this Book. Tell him how much
Mr. Freedom loves him and then demonstrate that love by being
a good friend to him right there in the prison. Remind him that
his stay in the city of Anytown is only temporary, and that it will
not be long before he will leave Anytown and travel to other
places in the land of Eternal Existence where no pain, no suffering, and no giants exist. Let him know that how he thinks and
acts right now in prison may determine what life will be like for
him later on in the other cities of Eternal Existence. So encourage him to spend his time here wisely. Rather than gripe, complain, or give up, suggest that he pass this information on to the
person sitting on the other side of him.

At first, Anyone didn't do anything. He simply wallowed in self-
pity, wondering what he had done to deserve this. Then one day, he
decided to go ahead and try what the Book suggested and turned to
the man sitting to his right side, Mr. Companion. They talked about
their suffering and how Mr. Pain had captured each of them. Anyone
shared some of the passages from the Book with Mr. Companion. To
Anyone's surprise, he forgot briefly about the pain he was in and even
that he was in prison. If the conversation provided only distraction, at
least it made him forget his pain for a short while and made him feel
less alone. Why not get to know the person on his left side, too, and
encourage his new friend to do the same?

So each of them began talking with prisoners near them. In this
way, the prisoners in that particular room got to know one another
and were soon planning a way to escape. Simply planning their escape, however, gave the prisoners hope and gave them something to
focus on. Some of the prisoners eventually escaped and others did
not. Nevertheless, for everyone who got involved in this activity, the
time in Mr. Pain's prison was a little easier.

Learning that Mr. Freedom was interested in their welfare, a number of the other prisoners called out to him for help. Some got to know
Mr. Freedom in a personal way for the first time in their lives. Some
read his Book for the first time. This changed how they saw themselves and how they saw others, including Mr. Freedom and Mr. Pain.

A few of these prisoners even began expressing sympathy for Mr. Pain, since the Book indicated that they should try to love even those who persecuted them. When they began to express concern for him, something wonderful happened. They started feeling better because they found their anger and resentment toward Mr. Pain lessen. They also found that their concern for him surprised and made Mr. Pain feel uneasy, so he spent less time taunting and torturing them because it wasn't much fun anymore.

Although Anyone was not one of the people who escaped from Mr. Pain's prison, he found that his life had new purpose and direction. He had more compassion for others in pain, much more than when he was living free. He also became a lot closer to Mr. Freedom during that time. Anyone began to like the person he had become in spite of his pain.

The End.

The next five chapters contain interviews with real people trapped in the prison of pain. These life stories have not been sugarcoated to comfort the reader; they tell events and feelings exactly as they were reported to me. Not selected specifically to illustrate any particular point, these are simply a sampling of patients and friends of mine with different chronic pain syndromes who agreed to be interviewed. They have been given fictitious names to encourage openness about their private experiences. Sufficient detail about their life histories has been provided so that you will get to know each person. Everyone was asked a similar set of questions about pain to discover how it affected their feelings about themselves, relationships with family, and their relationships with God; what they felt helped to relieve pain and what did not; how religious faith helped or did not help them to cope; what they learned from their pain; and what advice they had for others who also are suffering with pain.

Chapter 3

Back Pain—Bob's Story

Bob has been my patient for several years, and he is one of the reasons I decided to write this book. He is remarkably articulate in describing his pain, which has proven resistant to even the most advanced treatments, including multiple surgeries and large doses of narcotic pain relievers. He is a young man in the prime of his life, a family man with a wife and three children. He is a devout Christian with a deep and strong religious faith. Many under a similar burden would have ended their lives long ago. To be saddled with chronic, unrelenting pain at his age raises many questions. Although Bob's case is not really that unusual, it does provide a sobering picture of what it's like to live with chronic pain.

DR. KOENIG: When and where were you born?

BOB: I was born August 29, 1959, in Durham, North Carolina, right over here at Duke hospital.

DR. KOENIG: What was it like growing up for you?

BOB: I grew up in a home with a single parent. My father was in the picture, but he didn't live with us. My three sisters have a different father than I have. So I grew up with a mother who worked two jobs and supported four children.

DR. KOENIG: Did you have much while you were growing up—I mean, material things?

BOB: No, we grew up poor. My mother did the best she could with what she had. We didn't starve, but we lived in—I guess you would call it subsidized housing. She worked at Erwin Mills, a cotton mill located just off Main and Ninth Streets in Durham. She worked first shift there during the day, and took care of us and my invalid grandmother when she got home at night.

DR. KOENIG: How much schooling did you complete, and what kind of job or life aspirations did you have after you got out?

BOB: I graduated from high school. I wanted to be self-employed. I wanted to go ahead, before I was married, and make enough money to . . . I actually wanted to move to the coast. I loved the ocean so I wanted to move down to the coast and buy a motel, small, you know, twenty-five or thirty units, and just run a motel on the coast. That's what I was striving for.

DR. KOENIG: What was your first job?

BOB: My mother had a cousin who just opened up a 7-Eleven store in the neighborhood, four or five blocks up the street. He hired me that summer when I was about, I don't know, eight years old. All I did was sweep floors and separate drink bottles. And fill up bags of ice and stuff like that for a dollar an hour. Next, I got a paper route about the same time and did that for four years. When I was about eleven or twelve, I got a job working over on Driver Street at a place called Lynnett's Restaurant. I worked there pretty much full-time during the summers.

DR. KOENIG: What did you do after that?

BOB: My next job was at the Village Inn Pizza Parlor when I was sixteen. I learned the trade from the two guys who owned the store. I made pizzas and spaghetti and manicotti and ravioli. I did that about two years. When I worked there I was actually working three jobs. I worked at the pizza place, at a Buy Quick store part-time, and at a third job part-time, so I was working six days a week. I always arranged it so I could work every night through the week.

DR. KOENIG: Once you got out of high school, what did you do then?

BOB: I got a job at the A&P Supermarket while I was in high school, in my junior year, and I worked there too, along with the other jobs at the pizza place and at Buy Quick. The job at A&P lasted until 1986 when my son was born. I stayed there about thirteen years. My official title was a stock clerk. I started out working in produce, and moved from there to the grocery department. I ran a cash register, unloaded trucks, and ended up working in frozen foods, ordering all the frozen food for the store. In early 1987, I froze my retirement and left A&P. I had a daughter by my wife from her previous marriage, and when we had my son, my wife said, "You're never around. All you do is eat and sleep here." So I went ahead and gave that job up because I was working from 7:00 a.m. to 5:00 p.m. for the city of Durham and from 5:00 p.m. to 12:00 midnight at A&P.

DR. KOENIG: How long, then, did you work for the city of Durham?

BOB: I worked for the city from April 1978 until January 1999, and officially "retired" in September 1999, because of my back, and haven't worked since.

DR. KOENIG: When did you first get injured and how?

BOB: I got injured—I think it was October 1994. I was working for the city of Durham's waste management [sanitation] department. I had seven crews of people working for me—seven drivers and two collectors with each driver, so I had twenty-one people to supervise. One of the drivers called me on the radio and told me that his truck had broken down way out on Highway 54 and Highway 751, which would have been almost an hour drive from the office in a garbage truck. And he said, "I have to have another truck." Since it was late in the day, I told him that while we were waiting on the wrecker I would go out, find another truck, and bring it to him.

    The type of truck that we drove was built strangely. They didn't have a big hood on the front of the truck. The radiator, where you put the antifreeze, was on the back of the truck. I checked the antifreeze on one of the available trucks in the yard and it was low, so I got some and put it in. You had to climb up on the back of the truck to get to the motor. I've done it hundreds of times, if not thousands. I climbed up there and apparently spilled some of the antifreeze on the hood. As I started to climb down, my foot slipped out from under me, and I fell off the side of the truck. I didn't hit the ground, but caught myself on a hand railing the guys use to hold onto the truck. It snapped me hard, and the pain in my back started to bother me immediately.

DR. KOENIG: That was the first time you experienced back pain, in the fall of 1994, correct?

BOB: Yes, sir, it is.

DR. KOENIG: And you continued to work despite the pain?

BOB: I did. My supervisor was standing on the platform that day when I was taking the truck out, and he saw me fall. He asked me if I was okay, and I told him, "I think I just pulled a muscle or something." I went ahead and got the truck ready to go out, took the truck out to the fellows, and switched trucks with them. I had the other truck towed back in, went back to my office, and went back to work, and probably worked an hour or so. We're up and down a lot in our offices, answering the radios, on the computers and things. I got to the point where every time I got up my back was hurting really bad and pain was shooting down my leg.

DR. KOENIG: Prior to that injury were you in pretty good health?

BOB: I was never sick. I rarely had pain or anything.

DR. KOENIG: How many days each year did you usually take off from work for sickness?

BOB: I almost never missed work or took sick time. If I missed any at all it would be like one day a year. When I left my job at the city, I had almost a thousand hours sick time coming to me, and you accumulate those at a rate of six hours a month. So, I hadn't been sick for a long time.

DR. KOENIG: Now, when was your first surgery and how did it turn out?

BOB: My first surgery was in October 1994. I had a decompression done by a neurosurgeon who was very highly recommended. But the surgery didn't help. I still had problems.

DR. KOENIG: So you continued to have pain until a second surgery?

BOB: I had that one in February of 1996. I had a lower back fusion, and started having pain again soon after the surgery. I had trouble walking and was experiencing pain down the leg and into the foot. At first, for maybe two weeks, I thought everything was okay. I actually felt like I was getting better, and then the pain returned and has been there ever since.

DR. KOENIG: What limitations does your pain put on your life?

BOB: I really and truly don't know where to start. It stops me from spending a lot of time with my family, like going to amusement parks or the theaters. I'm not able to sit. I can't sit or stand for long periods of time. Even in the grocery store, if I had to stand in a long line, which is going to be over twenty minutes, I start immediately having problems. I can make it, and I can do it, but if I do it, I pay for it when I get home. What I mean by "paying for it" is the pain intensifies so much it literally makes me sick to my stomach.

DR. KOENIG: Describe the course of your pain during the day and the night. Go over a typical day. Do you wake up with pain? How does it restrict you in different ways?

BOB: When I wake up, sometimes I don't have pain right away. When I sit up, however, the pain is automatically there. As long as I'm lying flat when I wake up, most of the time I'm OK. On a morning like this morning, I had pain before I woke up. It woke me up.

DR. KOENIG: Go on . . .

BOB: I feel like once I get up, I'm really stiff. I get locked up in the back—meaning I can't flex and move good. It takes a few minutes to walk around and get going, and so I get up and usually fix a cup of coffee. I'll go outside and see my dogs. And I'll come back in the house and sit down for a while in my recliner. We homeschool our kids, so I do that.

DR. KOENIG: What about showers and getting dressed?

BOB: I usually take my shower at night, and so when I get up in the morning I just go ahead and get dressed. A lot of times I have trouble putting on my socks. Before I got hurt I was about one hundred forty pounds lighter than I am now, so of course the extra weight does not help. It hurts to try to bend your leg and bend your back to get your socks on. Clipping your toenails is a major task because you cannot flex your back to see what you are doing.

DR. KOENIG: Is it hard to put on your shoes?

BOB: It's not that hard, Dr. Koenig, but it does hurt because of having to bend my back when I'm sitting. It hurts to pull the leg up and get the shoe on the foot. They did give me some kind of device when I had the last surgery. It's like a long shoehorn that helps you put your foot in the shoe. And they gave me some shoestrings that were elastic so that you could slide your shoe onto your foot. After a while they break and pop out, so you're back to square one again.

DR. KOENIG: The pain starts in the morning, once you get up. Does it stick with you through the day?

BOB: Yes. It will subside for a while, and then intensifies again, depending on how much activity I'm doing. I'm always conscious of what I'm doing, and how much I'm doing, and how long I'm going to be gone when I leave my home. Because in physical therapy, I was trained, you can make it through an activity if you have rest periods. But if you push all the way through to the end, you'll just exhaust yourself. At this time of year, for example, mowing the grass is a major task. It's major. I have to stop three or four times and come in the house and rest—just mowing the grass.

DR. KOENIG: And that's a riding lawn mower, right?

BOB: Yes. I have a riding mower and a push mower. We have a small hill in front of our house, and so I have to mow the grass on the bank with the push mower. I actually feel better pushing the mower than riding the mower because sitting down and going out across the yard is actually worse on my back.

DR. KOENIG: When you sit down at night, say to watch TV, what is it like?

BOB: I have a recliner that I sit in. My daughter last night asked me why my toes were pulled up under each other. My toes will start drawing and pulling in like somebody with a bad case of rheumatoid arthritis. The toes pull up involuntarily under each other in the evening, especially if I've been busy during the day. I have sharp pains in the hips shooting down the back of the leg. Where the toe joints are connected to the foot itself, it feels like they're being heated by a butane lighter. I feel a tremendous amount of pressure in the lower back down below the belt line. It's always below the belt line. It feels like I have two handles on each side of my spine, and somebody who weighs about a hundred pounds is standing on the handles. It feels like my spine is being compressed.

DR. KOENIG: Have medications eased your pain? Narcotic pain relievers, for example?

BOB: No. The only thing that has helped my pain at all is the TENS unit [transcutaneous nerve stimulator]. I guess it diverts your mind from the pain, so to speak. I've actually found it more beneficial for my feet than for my back. I guess it's because of the thickness and large mass of my body, and where the nerves are in my back, that the TENS just does not produce enough vibration to get down to it. But in my toes, when my toes are burning real bad, it really helps.

DR. KOENIG: Now when you go to bed at night, how does the pain affect your falling asleep and staying asleep?

BOB: I don't stay asleep, that's the problem. I usually go to bed about 11, 11:30 every night. I try to go to sleep without a sleeping pill, but if I take it [Ambien], I'm usually asleep by about 12:30. By 3:00 a.m., though, I'm awake again.

DR. KOENIG: You're having pain when you both fall asleep and wake up?

BOB: The pain is with me almost constantly. There's very little time in my life since I've been hurt that I do not have pain.

DR. KOENIG: The surgery didn't help your pain at all?

BOB: It did not. I've also had spinal nerve blocks, but they didn't help either.

DR. KOENIG: Have any alternative medicine treatments, natural substances, or anything in that category helped your pain?

BOB: I've tried a heat wrap on my back that helps when the pain is real bad. It's a thing you put in the microwave, and it has some kind of corn husk that you heat up . . . it's like a heating pad. I've also used magnets on my back. That helps at times. What I've found to be most beneficial, and I don't have one but I noticed it when we've traveled, is a whirlpool or hot tub. Sometimes when I'm really stiff we go to our neighbor's house, and he has an outdoor swimming pool. In the water, with that much less resistance, it helps everything out. I walk back and forth in the pool, you know, and let the kids play.

DR. KOENIG: What about anything that you've actually taken—pills, organic preparations, or vitamins?

BOB: I tried some pills from a health food store that are supposed to get all of the impurities out of your body. It's called Flora Force. It didn't help. It cost like twenty-five bucks.

DR. KOENIG: Have you tried anything else?

BOB: The one thing I tried that helped a little bit was from Wellspring Grocery. It's called White Tiger Balm. It's like BenGay rub, so to speak. It's a medicine that's made, I guess, in China. I haven't had any in awhile, but the lady that worked with me after I had the surgery—the physical therapist that specializes in rehabilitation of people with back surgery—she recommended it. It's like a heat penetrating lotion. It will help for a while, for an hour or so, and then it diminishes. But at least it helps a little bit.

DR. KOENIG: On to another topic, now. How has the pain affected you personally, how has it affected your feelings about yourself?

BOB: I feel like the pain has taken my life away. I don't know how to explain it any other way. You know, when you're in so much pain and you're trying to escape from the pain and you cannot escape, you feel like you are trapped, and you feel like there is no way out. You try not to think about the pain all the time. You try to think about more pleasant things, but the pain is always there and is always pressing in. And any moment you have any freedom from it, you feel like, "Oh God, if I do this, what am I going to feel like later? If I do this today, am I going to hurt tonight? Since I don't have much pain right now, is this activity going to intensify the pain?" It makes you very timid because you're afraid to do anything. The next thing you do could cause pain. Anywhere you go or anyway you act, you can't predict what might happen. You always have that thought in the back of your mind saying, "Well, if I do this, am I going to pay for it?"

DR. KOENIG: How does that make you feel about yourself?

BOB: It makes me feel less of a man, because you feel like you can't do things that other men can do. It takes away some of your manhood. I don't know how to explain it other than that.

DR. KOENIG: How has the pain affected your family life?

BOB: We don't have any what you call quality time. There's not a whole lot I can do, Dr. Koenig. My son wants to play baseball, and I do go out with him sometimes and try to play. But I just can't play for over about fifteen minutes. I mean, you know, I pitch him the ball, he hits the ball, and the ball is on the ground. Either he's going to run and go get the ball and get tired, or I've got to bend down there and pick it up somehow. And so we really and truly don't do a whole lot. Now he does like to fish. And we do have a small boat that I try to take him fishing in from time to time. But other than that, we don't really do much. I feel bad about that.

DR. KOENIG: How has the pain affected your relationship with your wife?

BOB: Well, we don't really do much together either. We don't go out anywhere or do anything. I mean, you're married, of course, but you know how when you first started dating you did a lot of things together? You're in love and everywhere you go and everything you do, you want your spouse or girlfriend with you. But now it's like, you know, we don't do anything outside of the church. We're working this week at vacation Bible school, or trying to. I'm trying to. We left early last night. But we don't really do a whole lot together. We don't go out to eat anymore. And we don't go to the movies because I can't sit that long.

DR. KOENIG: How do you think this pain has affected the way your wife views you? How your wife looks at you?

BOB: I know she knows I'm in pain sometimes, but sometimes I wonder if she thinks, "Are you putting on?" You know, "Are you really feeling this bad, or are you just wanting a little sympathy for your problem?" I don't want nobody to have any sympathy for me. I've always been self-sufficient. The Lord has blessed me with being able to do what I need to do. I do not like to ask for help. I want to be the one *giving* the help, but I don't like to be the one receiving it. I feel like that makes me less of a man if you need a whole lot of help to do something.

One night last week I went outside to feed the dogs and my leg gave away on me and it threw me out on the carport. I laid out there about twenty minutes trying to get my wits about me and get back up to the house. My wife comes through the door and panics. She called the rescue squad, and it made me mad. It really and truly did. I told her, I said, "Don't call them. I don't want them out here." While she was talking with the 911 operator, I was doing everything I could to get up so that she would stop. It took all I had to get up, to just stand up and be able to get my legs up under me. When I came into the house, I told her that I'd refuse to go to the hospital. I just wouldn't go.

DR. KOENIG: Did the paramedics show up?

BOB: She still had them on the phone and had them on the way, and I told her, I said, "If they come out here, I'm not going." I said, "Cancel it, because I'm not going to the hospital just because I fell down the doorstep." And so when the paramedics arrived they helped me into the bed. It took about thirty minutes because once I sat down, my back went into bad cramps and spasms and I couldn't lie on the bed. It took a while to get me into the bed. But it really and truly embarrassed me.

DR. KOENIG: Let's talk about how the pain has affected you spiritually.

BOB: You ask God, "Why me? What did I do?" You feel like you're being punished for some sin you committed in your life. You know, we all commit sin every day we open our eyes. But you feel like, "God, are you punishing me for something I did, way back when I was out there at the nightclubs and chasing the women? Are you punishing me for that? Are you punishing me for something I didn't do, a calling I didn't pursue? Did I not do what I was supposed to do and be obedient?" So, you know, God is a God of forgiveness, and he doesn't like to see his children suffer. But then again, on the other hand, you say, "Lord, why me?" I mean, you think about that a lot in detail. And you read Scripture. A lot of times I'll sit down at night to read the Bible, and I'll say, "Show me why I've got this." You'll open the Bible up and your eye will be right on it, and the scripture will say, "My grace is sufficient for thee." Or something like that. And it's like the Lord is telling me, "This is a burden that you're going to have to carry. I carried the cross and your sin, and you've got to carry this." If there's a reason for it, if it's to glorify Him, then I'll carry it until the day I die.

DR. KOENIG: What other questions do you ask God about concerning your pain?

BOB: I guess I ask him, "Why do I have to live with it?" I guess that's the only thing I ask him. "Why do I have to live with the pain? What is it that you want me to learn from this in my Christian walk?" I like to see, I guess, answers in the flesh. "If you want me to do this and you want me to have this pain, then make it very plain what you expect from me." Just thinking about it sometimes confuses me even more. I want it like Moses. I want it written out like God did with the Ten Commandments.

DR. KOENIG: What is it you want written out?

BOB: That if this is my life journey, if I must deal with pain the rest of my life, then I'd like God to show me why I have to deal with it. Then I could handle the journey that I've got to take. I have a high tolerance for pain. I can take a lot. I really and truly can. I could before I was hurt. I played football in high school. I've always been the type that could take a lot of pain. But sometimes now, I feel like I'm at the breaking point with this pain.

DR. KOENIG: What could friends or church members do to help you with the pain?

BOB: They could pray for me. As far as I know, that's the only thing they could do that would help. Of course, when stuff happens at home, if you had somebody that could help you do something, of course that would help. For instance, a while back the pump gave out in my well. We're on well water. I can't pull that pump out of the well now. It's down about a hundred feet in the ground. And so I had to have a well company, a plumber, come over here and pull it out. Before I was hurt, I would have pulled that rascal out of there, got a pump, hooked it up myself, and put it back. I can't do that now.

DR. KOENIG: Would it help if people offered to help you do some practical things that you need done?

BOB: Yes, it would. I don't know, maybe not. . . . It bothers me when they do that because it makes me feel less of a man.

DR. KOENIG: Do you ever ask them to help you?

BOB: No, I don't. My wife will ask them to help me. She will sometimes say, "Can you help him do so and so," or "Would you ask him if he'd like some help?" But in general, I don't usually ask people. Now I have, since you and me talked awhile back, started to ask for help. Sometimes I had things that were just impossible for me to do, so I have asked people to help me do those things.

DR. KOENIG: How do you feel when your wife asks people to do things for you?

BOB: It embarrasses me.

DR. KOENIG: Tell me why.

BOB: Well, you see, I guess it all goes back to how I was raised. My mother taught us if you wanted something, the only way you're going to get it honestly is to work for it. You know, God gives you a body and gives you the strength to do what you need to do with your life. You can't go out there and move a mountain, of course, but, you know, my mother taught us to be independent. Because she said you can have what you want in life, but you have to get it on your own by hard work and determination and perseverance.

DR. KOENIG: Now, tell me, what should church friends *not* do?

BOB: I don't want sympathy from them. I don't want anybody to feel sorry for me. This is *my* problem. I feel in a certain way that I caused the problem I've got because I fell off the truck. Nobody pushed me off the truck. A drunk driver didn't hit me. I don't want any sympathy from anybody. I just want them to, you know . . .

DR. KOENIG: To what?

BOB: I want them not to look at me like I'm handicapped, like I'm crippled. I'm dealing with the pain the very best that I can. I don't want them to treat me any differently than they would other people.

DR. KOENIG: What else could church friends do—or not do?

BOB: I really and truly don't know. I guess one thing that bothers me more than anything is that we don't have any family to watch our kids when my wife and I want to go out. So if the church were to start, I guess, a children's night, where parents could get out. You know, like I volunteer this Friday night, you volunteer next Friday night. Even if it's just for two hours, just to give the adults that have children, including me and my wife, time to get out and be by themselves. Not everyone has parents who live nearby that they can leave their children with. See, my mother has passed away, and my wife's father has passed away. My wife's family lives in Florida. My dad is not able to keep my children. And we have nobody else.

DR. KOENIG: Anything else that church people could do to help?

BOB: A support group at the church for people with chronic pain would help. We have support groups in our church. I'm involved in a group that goes to the hospital and visits the sick. I say to them, "I'm from the men's ministry at the church. I've come out to see how you are doing. I'd like to pray for you. Is there anything that you need? Does your family need dinners at night brought to them while you're getting straightened out? Is there some work you need done at your house that the men's ministry can help with?" We ask that and we're sincere about it. If they have a need, we try to identify it and fill the need.

DR. KOENIG: So if there were a support group like that for people with chronic pain, it would help?

BOB: Yeah, I think it really would. It would help.

DR. KOENIG: How might they offer help in a way that you would accept it?

BOB: I guess if they did it churchwide, then I wouldn't think that they were doing it just for me. Then everyone could benefit from it. And I wouldn't personally feel like they're saying, "Well, you know Bob's back is hurt. We feel obligated to go over there and help. You know, we feel obligated because he is one of the deacons. You know, we need to go over there and help him out. I really and truly don't want to go, but you know, we ought to go because we don't want people in the church talking about it." If it were churchwide, everybody would be eligible for it, not just Bob.

DR. KOENIG: Let's switch over from church friends to family. What could your family do to help you with your pain? What could your wife, what could your kids do?

BOB: My family members don't understand what kind of pain I go through because I hide it a lot.

DR. KOENIG: So what could they do to help?

BOB: I hate to say it like this, but if they could *feel* what I'm going through—but I wouldn't wish that on my worst enemy. People don't understand, Dr. Koenig, until they've had it. I've heard people in the church tell me, "Man, I sprained my back last week, and I can imagine what you're going through." And I'm thinking to myself, "No, you can't." And they're saying, "My back hurt me so bad I had to take two days off work, but you know, the doctor gave me some pills and I feel a whole lot better." You can't really know what I'm going through because you haven't walked in my shoes. You haven't had pain twenty-four hours a day for years and years. If I could reach in there and pop my spine out of my back and I knew it would stop the pain, I'd do it in a second.

DR. KOENIG: So your family could try harder to understand what it is like to have this kind of pain all the time?

BOB: One of the things my children could probably do is to be more understanding. For instance, my youngest daughter, eight-year-old Lisa, wants to go swimming all the time. And some days I just don't feel like going, and she doesn't understand that. She gets mad and pouts because Daddy won't take her swimming. And my boy is saying, "You don't want to go out in the yard and play ball with me. You don't want to take me fishing. You don't want to take me to the mall. You don't want to do nothing with me. You don't want to take me to the movies. So and so goes to the movies. So and so goes here and there. How come you can't take me?"

DR. KOENIG: Continue . . .

BOB: I mean, you know, I hate to unload like this, but it's the truth. And my wife doesn't say anything. A lot of times she'll get up and get ready to go to the mall. And I'll say, "Where are you going?" And she'll say, "Well, I want to go out to the mall, or just walk around. I'm trying to shop a little for Christmas, birthdays, or something." And I'll say, "I'll go with you." And she'll say "Well, you must be in a lot of pain today. I know you don't feel like going so I'll just run. . . . I'm not going to be gone long," or "I'm going to be gone long, and I know how you're going to feel. So I'm just going to go ahead by myself." Or her and my oldest daughter will go. So there you are and you feel like you were left out again. You're at home because of your pain.

DR. KOENIG: What could they do specifically in those circumstances to help you feel better about it?

BOB: I think probably to include me. Even though I know I'm going to hurt, I've got to feel like in my heart and mind that I'm benefiting part of society. You cannot live your life sitting at home saying, "Oh, God, my back's hurting so bad. My leg's hurting so bad." I still have to feel productive. It's depressing when you're at home, and you're by yourself all day long. You don't have anybody coming around, any of your friends, because everybody's working.

It's the same thing when the church goes on overnight camping trips. Our Sunday school classes are going out to Falls Lake. I mean, I live five minutes from the lake. The church goes on boating activities, and they go up to the lake and water-ski and stuff like that. Can I go? No, I cannot go. Likewise, my son goes on trips with the youth. And they go out camping and do lots of fun things. Can I go? No, I cannot, because I can't lay on the ground in a sleeping bag. Can I go with them when they go to New Hampshire? They're going up there to start a new church this week. They'll also go around witnessing in the neighborhoods. Can I do that? No, I cannot. I can't handle that— I can't walk from door to door talking to people. Would I like to? You bet. I would love to do it. And so every time they go somewhere and do something, I'm left out again. Not intentionally, but my pain keeps me from participating in those things.

DR. KOENIG: What I hear you saying is that you would like your family to include you even if it involves some pain, but to be respectful of your limitations. What else?

BOB: They should not feel sorry for me. They should be willing to understand what I'm going through when I do ask for help. Like washing the dishes, and simple stuff, like taking out the garbage ... When we go to the grocery store, and the dog food needs to be brought in, I say, "Can you put the dog food under the counter?" My little one says, "Oh, Daddy, I don't want to do that." Well, we got a certain place under the counter where we keep dog food, and you have to squat down there, or kneel down, and it's almost on the floor level. We keep only dog food in there. Well, you get in there and straighten up whatever's in there so you can stack the dog food neatly, but I have trouble doing that. Since my wife works and I'm at home during the day, I usually try to cook dinner—but I can't do everything. Do you want me to do all the cooking and the washing and the whole nine yards that needs doing around the house? And then lay in the bed at night and cry because I hurt so bad that I feel like I'm going out of my mind? I'd just like them to be more responsible as far as being attentive to what needs to be done around the house. To be more helpful with the household chores.

DR. KOENIG: Anything else that your wife should or should not do?

BOB: I don't want her—as I'll reiterate, I don't want her to feel sorry for me. This is a cross that I'm going to have to carry on my own.

DR. KOENIG: How do you want her to treat you?

BOB: Treat me like any other man, you know. I want to be treated like any other man. If something needs to be done, don't just say, "Well, I tried to do it because I didn't think you could do it." At least give me the opportunity, let me answer, rather than make a decision for me. I know where my limitations and boundaries are.

DR. KOENIG: So let you establish those boundaries, not establish them for you?

BOB: Right.

DR. KOENIG: OK, on to another subject. What has helped you the most in coping emotionally with your pain?

BOB: Prayer.

DR. KOENIG: And what does prayer do?

BOB: Prayer gives me a way to release, to talk to God about my problems, and to ask for help from the spiritual realm.

DR. KOENIG: And how does prayer affect your pain?

BOB: Well, maybe it doesn't affect the severity of the pain as much as it affects your attitude toward the pain. You know that God is omnipotent and omnipresent—He's always there. He can hear everybody's prayer at the same time, and He is able to heal you even if no one else can. He hears every prayer you ask, and you know that you are His child, so if anybody can help you, God can.

DR. KOENIG: Knowing that, what does that do for you?

BOB: It gives a sense of relief to know that there's somebody who can hear you and can help you. If anybody can help you, He can. Jesus felt what pain is like on the cross, for us.

DR. KOENIG: So prayer is the thing that really helps you the most—talking to God?

BOB: Yes.

DR. KOENIG: Anything else? What's the second most important thing that helps you to cope?

BOB: To be able to just lay down and relax, get off my feet and stretch out and let my back relax. You know what I'm saying? Physically relax.

DR. KOENIG: And that helps with the pain?

BOB: Yeah.

DR. KOENIG: Can you see any good in your pain?

BOB: The other week I went to see this couple from our church. We were doing visitation. They asked me, they said, "How's your back doing? You don't look like you're hurting today." And I said, "Well, in all honesty, I hide a lot of the pain." And they said, "Well, it's good that you can get out and visit other people, because if they've had a hip replacement or whatever, and they see you out there doing things, they'll think, if he can do it, I can do it." I guess there is some good in your being able to encourage other people with health problems, help them understand that there is life even if a person experiences a lot of pain.

DR. KOENIG: So, the good in your pain is that it might give you understanding of what other people are going through, so that you can act as a role model—demonstrating that you can live with pain and have a life.

BOB: Right.

DR. KOENIG: Can you see any purpose in your pain?

BOB: No, I cannot. I don't see any purpose in it at all. It's like, as we talked about, the cross I'm to bear.

DR. KOENIG: Say a little bit more about that.

BOB: The Lord never promised us that it would be easy when we became Christians. A lot of times I look at Job in the Bible. Job was a righteous man, and was without sin in God's eyes, so to speak. Not completely without sin, of course he was born into sin. When God and the devil began talking, the Lord said, "Have you considered my servant Job? He is righteous and holy." And the devil said, "If you'll allow me to take his health from him, then surely he will curse you and turn his back on you." Despite all the pain Job went through, he never did that. Even his friends, some of them, the men of that time, when they saw him they just sat down and cried. They couldn't believe the type of pain that he was suffering. But God knew what the final outcome would be. No matter how much the devil did to Job, and no matter how much pain Job suffered, God knew that somewhere down the road his pain would end and everything would be restored to him.

DR. KOENIG: Have you grown psychologically or spiritually as a result of your pain?

BOB: Yes, because I used to think that people who complained a lot with pain were putting on a whole lot, that it couldn't hurt that bad. You know, that it wasn't really all that bad. And I didn't have any sympathy for them. Now, since I've walked in their shoes, I realize that maybe I was judgmental in a lot of things I thought about those people. I'm not as judgmental as I was, because I know there's pain that's actually crippling pain. And if people are dealing with it the very best they can, that's all they can do. I mean they can't heal themselves.

DR. KOENIG: Has your pain caused you to become closer to God?

BOB: Very much so. I feel like that's the only person that I have that I can really and truly count on. Because you figure no one else really understands you like God does, and God understands everything you're going through. And he knows there's a purpose for you going through it. When I get home to heaven, the first question I'm going to ask is, "Why? Why me?" And he's going to probably say, "Why not you? If my son did all of this, why not you? What's the big deal with you taking it?" And I still won't know my answer.

DR. KOENIG: What kind of advice would you have for other people like yourself with chronic pain? That's the last question.

BOB: If you are a Christian, pray that you can be a witness and that whatever pain you have and whatever you go through, that in some way you can bring glory to God.

Follow-Up

Several months after this interview, Bob reported that he was handling his pain better. The pain had not reduced in intensity, still hardly ever dropping below a five on a zero to ten scale and often approaching nine or ten. However, he indicated that he was doing better. Why? Bob said that he had "accepted" the pain, and had begun to talk with other sufferers about their pain: not immediately saying, "I know what you're going through," but listening to them, detecting common struggles, and then identifying specifically with those struggles. In this way he had created a small support group of others in pain who could talk to each other and help each other get through it.

He brought up another important point. He said that people in pain are in many ways similar to alcoholics or drug addicts. In each case, something is threatening to take over the person's life. To successfully get back in control of his life, Bob said he needed to help himself. "You need to help yourself," he said. "You've got to make decisions and do things that will lead toward your healing." Of course, Bob was quick to note that you've also got to recognize that you can't do it all by yourself. Partnering with God and with others, then, seems essential.

Chapter 4

Headache Pain—Penny's Story

Penny is a middle-aged Christian woman who for nearly a decade has struggled with migraine headaches. She is married, has four children, and is a housewife. This chapter tells her story, focusing on a horrendous three-week period during which she was completely incapacitated with severe, recurrent headaches. The discussion will focus on how she felt and how it affected her activity, family, and spiritual life. Many of those who suffer from headaches will see similarities to their own stories in the pages ahead.

DR. KOENIG: When and where were you born?

PENNY: On the Eastern shore in Maryland on December 9, 1954.

DR. KOENIG: Tell me what it was like growing up?

PENNY: It was kind of mixed. The good part was my dad's job in the civil service that allowed us to spend many summers on the Eastern shore. When I was four, however, we moved to the middle of the Mojave Desert in California. I really enjoyed those summers on the Eastern shore and missed them after the move. The negative side was that my mother is bipolar and was the daughter of a man who was bipolar. My grandfather was an alcoholic, and she was an alcoholic, and being the daughter of an alcoholic bipolar who was in and out of hospitals for six to nine months at a time was kind of tough. Even when she was home, you didn't know if she was going to throw you a kiss or an ashtray when you walked in the door after school. These were difficult times, as you can imagine, but as an adult I feel like I'm pretty prepared to face a lot of things because of it.

DR. KOENIG: How much education did you have and what aspirations did you have after completing school?

PENNY: I have a bachelor of arts in liberal studies. I thought I'd be a children's librarian someday. I wanted something quiet and I absolutely loved children's books and loved reading out loud to children. But life . . . I got pregnant and had four children.

DR. KOENIG: What was the first job that you had after you completed school?

PENNY: I worked for a physician for seven years during the time that I was in school, and then when I graduated, I continued to work for him for awhile. But after I had two children that were crying at my legs, "Please don't leave me at day care," I just couldn't take it anymore and sort of had a burnout time, I guess you'd call it. And my husband said in six months I could resign. So I did that in 1986, and became mostly a full-time housewife.

DR. KOENIG: So you've been a housewife most of the time since you quit that job?

PENNY: When I first came back from the West, which would have been five years ago, I taught fourth grade at a local Christian school. You didn't have to be certified to teach there. You just had to have a college degree, and I had that and some other training that they needed, and certainly the Christian background. I worked for ten months teaching fourth grade. Then the school unfortunately went belly up, so a couple of years ago I started to substitute teach, which is what I'm still doing. Obviously up and down, but by the end of the school year I'm working five days a week.

DR. KOENIG: When and how did you meet your husband, Asim?

PENNY: Asim and I met by chance. I had only been a Christian for about nine months, and I'd wake up every morning praying, "God, give me a job. Can I do anything for you?" And I went back to my two-year college to pick up my associate degree—you know, you get a fake piece of paper at graduation and then you go back to get the real one. Well, I was in the office getting the real paper that said I had an associate degree, when I just bumped into him in the office and said, "Can I help you in any way?" I knew he was an unbeliever but I just thought maybe God might use me. And so I gave him my phone number and said, "If I can help you settle in, if there's anything I can do for you, give me a call." Well, he served Christ with me despite the fact that he was a nonbeliever. He did pray some and we had very similar values—aside from Christ. I was twenty-four and ready for a permanent relationship. So I said, "Is it okay, God? Oh good," and jumped in. We got married in 1978.

DR. KOENIG: How many children do you have and what are their ages?

PENNY: I have four. Brittany's almost nineteen, Jenny's sixteen, Michael is twelve, and Tommy is nine.

DR. KOENIG: When did you first experience headaches?

PENNY: It was when we lived in Durham, before we moved to Raleigh. I think it was before Tommy was born, so it was probably approximately nine years ago. I went to the doctor after the first headache because it was quite extreme and I had never had anything like it. I thought maybe I was going to have a stroke or something. This pain came up the left side of my neck and went across my head. It happened when I was alone, and I was really afraid. So I called a taxi to take me to the hospital. They did a spinal tap that was negative. While it's hard to remember, I know they didn't give me a shot or do anything special. Basically they referred me to a neurologist.

DR. KOENIG: How did your visit with the neurologist go?

PENNY: When I saw the neurologist, I took the three kids into the office with me. The guy was really snippy. He said, "Well, no wonder you have headaches. What are you, a Catholic?" I don't know why he had such a negative view toward children. But I knew that I wanted a fourth child, and when I read the package insert on the Inderal he'd prescribed, it said it might not be too good to be pregnant during the first trimester when taking that drug. I went back to him and I said, "You know, I don't think this is the drug for me because I know I want to get pregnant again." And he said, "Well, I just can't help you then." So he pretty much just dropped me.

DR. KOENIG: Did you seek further help?

PENNY: I went on, and every few months I would get one of these headaches. They were still similar to the first one, but not as severe. What I would do is lay down for five hours, and pray, or try so hard to just rest and lie really still and stay in the dark. At that time I didn't seek out other help. I never sought out migraine medication or anything. I did learn about some of the things that caused it. Obviously, you're a doctor, so I'm just going to come out and say it. I had coital headaches. Right before orgasm I would get them. I would moan out, "Oh God, my head." It would just go straight up and that was it, boy. It was over. And then I'd be down for five hours.

DR. KOENIG: Did anything else bring the headaches on?

PENNY: Yes. Like if Asim would have ring-around-the-collar, and I'd put soap on it and I'd take my thumbs and scrub out the ring, the force of pushing down would bring on a headache. Now I've tried to mock that, and people say that I do something with my face, and they think maybe I strain my jaw or something when I'm doing that, which might be bringing it on.

DR. KOENIG: So just straining to get the ring out, maybe through your facial expressions of exerting yourself, would bring it on?

PENNY: Exactly, and I've noticed something else that I do. This is so silly. Tommy pointed it out to me. Tommy is a clown and he watches people and he mocks them because he thinks it's funny and he's a little kid. Through him I realized something that I do that I wasn't even aware of until he did it. When I get excited about something, I'm like this little child. I'm like this giggly girl and I kind of squeeze my elbows to my breasts, you know, to my side, and I put my hands together like a little squirrel or something. And then I bear down with my face a little toward my chest, and I hold my breath, "Oh gosh! It's so exciting!" You know. I don't mean to. It just happens.

DR. KOENIG: When did it happen the last time?

PENNY: Remember the great snow of February 2000, when we got two feet in twenty-four hours? The first one occurred right before that, like two days before the snow. And snow is my very favorite, so I missed the entire time. I was so sad. I was down for maybe seven or eight hours. But this was an unusually difficult one, because there was absolutely no rest, no peace, and it was a lot more pain than I'd ever had. It was harder than even the first time. The first time I was scared because I'd never had anything like it. And then every few months I'd have one, but I'd say the pain was somewhere around three or four on a pain scale of zero to ten. But this last one was different—and it lasted for nearly three and one-half weeks.

DR. KOENIG: What was the pain like during that period?

PENNY: It went up to a ten. It was so bad I was truly challenged as a Christian. Had we a weapon in the house at the time, I'm very afraid of what I might have done. I'm not kidding. I'd already prayed everything and recited as many Scriptures as I could. I'd even gone back to my precollege years, and tried to remember every bit of yoga and meditation and other relaxation methods that I had learned. I tried to focus the pain beyond myself. I did everything I could think of, but nothing worked. I was sleep deprived. There would be ten-hour periods of extreme, excruciating pain, where there was no relief, no rest. I was taking a migraine medicine called Darvocet. I also took the new migraine medicines that they have on the television. You know, the expensive migraine medicine that they'll only give you three tablets at a time because of the insurance company [Midrin]. And I'd take one, and it would do absolutely nothing. Nothing touched it. That was just the first day.

DR. KOENIG: Did you call a doctor?

PENNY: I didn't call my doctor the first day, even though it was getting really bad. You have to realize, I didn't know it was going to get worse and worse. Because I'd had something like this before, and then after five hours I was okay. So the fact that this took three hours longer, and was a little more intense, I didn't know what was going to happen. So I was just being patient and trying to work through it, right? Well, then, I babied myself the next day since I really didn't feel back to myself. That was different than the other times. The other times, after five hours, I could get up and get back to my life. But that didn't happen after this one. I didn't feel right. Something wasn't right. So the second day, I just went kind of easy.

DR. KOENIG: Then what?

PENNY: The next morning, we woke up to that tremendous snow— eighteen to twenty-four inches, right? Well, since I'm a nut over snow, I walked outside. Asim was already out because he gets up a little earlier than me, and he was going to start to shovel, and I said, "Oh no, don't shovel yet. Let me get a camera." And I ran in, got the camera took a picture, and then I went, "Oh, I'm so excited," like I did when Tommy described it. And that was it. I had to drop the camera and run into the house. I grabbed a package of peas out of the freezer and ran upstairs, the whole time thinking, "I'm going to drop right here and lay, because it's too late. I've got the headache." It shot from the back of the left side of my head, and was like a monstrous hand squeezing my brain as hard as it could.

DR. KOENIG: What did you do then?

PENNY: I put the peas over my face, but I could smell that freezer smell, and it sickened me. And I was about to vomit. You know, I was just so sick. The pain was, I mean, it was going from an eight to a ten. Then I realized, "Oh Lord Jesus, I am trapped. If I'm having an aneurysm right now . . ." I mean, I'm not a person that typically, you know, I don't go overboard on stuff, but I thought, "Lord, I've never felt a pain like this in my life. This must not be a migraine. I must have a bleed." And I'm laying there thinking, "The EMS can't get to me. There are eighteen inches of snow in North Carolina. I am trapped. I am in this bed, and nobody can get to me, and I'm going to die of an aneurysm." At that point, I didn't want to die. I was thinking more about the kids. I wasn't sleep deprived yet, you know. I really wanted to survive, so I was in a fighting mode. But it was the longest ten hours of my life. I was useless. There was nothing I could do. Asim had to take care of everything around the house. Well, after ten hours of no sleep, no rest, no relief from the pain, it started to finally ease off. Now at this point, Asim did try to reach my doctor. They started calling things in, and he would pick them up. And I would take things every few hours to try to get relief, but nothing they gave me helped.

DR. KOENIG: So when did the headache finally stop?

PENNY: After several hours, it seemed to ease off. When I finally got through it, though, I still didn't feel right. I felt like I was walking on eggshells. Something wasn't normal with me. "I really better be careful," I thought, and was just like pulling myself through the day. I never got dressed. I moved around gently and carefully, not really doing anything, but lying down on the couch as much as I could because I was just pretty much afraid to move. When I got up the next morning, I said to myself, "Listen, girl, you haven't done anything around here now for five days. You have got to do something." My four children can mess up this house pretty badly. So I went into the kitchen, and somebody the night before had eaten hot dogs and gotten ketchup on the counter, and it had kind of dried. All I did was take the sponge, and I pushed down hard enough to try to remove that ketchup, and there it came again, right up the left side. I was down again. I was down for seven or eight hours. That was it. I was in bed. I was useless. At this point, I'm thinking, "Oh, great. I'm three migraines in. Asim's been serving me. And now he's going to come home and I'm down again. There's nothing I can do." I couldn't even use the phone to call my doctor. I couldn't even really move my mouth. Some of the time, if I tried to move my mouth, I would get sick to my stomach. You know, I'd get so nauseated.

DR. KOENIG: Boy, that must have been hard.

PENNY: It was so hard. You know, some of the time there just wasn't anybody that could help me. Or nobody that knew I was in trouble. There might be people in the house, but they just didn't know I was in trouble and I couldn't communicate that. One particular time, I picked up my phone and dialed zero, and I said, "Operator, I'm very sick, and I need my daughter downstairs to come bring me some medicine." And I said, "Can you please ring my house?" And she did it. She somehow rang my own house. So Jenny picked up the phone, and I said, "Jenny, honey, come help me." Then I got through. It was happening, you know, like every other day. I'd have a day of uncomfortable reprieve, maximum two days, but where I wasn't really functioning. And I was just being a bum basically, so there was guilt on top of . . .

DR. KOENIG: Because you were afraid to do anything.

PENNY: Oh, I was terrified to do anything, because, I just knew I couldn't take the pain anymore. I knew I'd be completely useless again if the headache came back. At least now I could tell somebody else, "Hey, things are getting out of hand. Please pick this up." But if I'm on my back, I couldn't say anything to anybody. It was such a hard time.

DR. KOENIG: What about your doctor?

PENNY: He had a really full schedule and couldn't see me. He referred me to this doctor, who I won't name. But it's a woman with the least compassion of any human being I've ever met. She didn't know me. I don't know how much of my chart she read. But she made up her mind that I was somebody who must be abusing pain medications. I know that there are people that like pain medications and will go to the ER just to get them, saying "Oh, my head hurts." I have never, would never do that. I'm a Christian. I hate drugs. I don't like anything that makes me feel any different than I already feel. I just wanted a rest. I just wanted something to make the pain stop long enough to let me sleep a few hours. Even though I'd sleep a little bit, I'd never get any rest. During this three-and-a-half-week period, I really became sleep deprived.

DR. KOENIG: How did things change as you became more and more sleep deprived?

PENNY: I feel like my walk with the Lord was challenged because as I got more and more worn out I was thinking, "Lord, I know you can hear me. But what's happening? You said you wouldn't give me more than I can bear, but I'm almost there, Lord. I've had almost as much as I can bear. I just don't know how much longer . . ." See, I had four C-sections. My first baby came three months early. I pulled my pole down the hall the second my feet would touch the floor, despite having an epidural. With Jenny, my second baby, I had another epidural. Unfortunately, they punctured my dura [membrane surrounding the spinal cord] with the epidural needle, resulting in a severe spinal headache. And there was nothing ordered for pain, so I just had to tough it out. So I'm no sissy. I can take pain. I get cortisone shots in the bottom of my foot for my plantar fasciitis and I just pretty much sit there.

DR. KOENIG: Sounds like you have a pretty high pain threshold.

PENNY: I really can take pain, but this was just beyond my mortal limits, you know? I couldn't try any longer. I was at God's mercy, but I felt like I wasn't getting any mercy. And that's horrible to say, but I was just exhausted. I felt like, "Lord, no more. I can't take anymore." And this doctor was being such a poo-poo. So finally, my next door neighbor, who is a physician, got on the phone with this woman and said, "Listen, I've known Penny for four years. Some people fake migraines to get heavy-duty pain medication, but you've got the wrong picture here. Please, at least make a referral to a neurologist or somebody. Let's do something."

DR. KOENIG: Did that help?

PENNY: Well, they brought me in because I had another one in the meantime. And when I was having this other one, it was again a ten. I started taking a wet, dark brown washcloth and covering my eyes with it. But I was having so much pain that I involuntarily had started to rub my face with the washcloth. I rubbed I don't know how many layers of skin off my face. It looked like I was wind-burned. I didn't know what I was doing. And the sound . . . I could hear this sound coming out of me. I sounded like an animal. I can't mock it because I don't really remember it. I forget what it sounded like, but I know that there was this noise coming out of me that I wasn't trying to make. I was aware of making it. I could hear it. But it was like I couldn't help it.

DR. KOENIG: What did the doctor say?

PENNY: When I finally got into the doctor's office, she said if Asim would go down to the pharmacy and get some Darvon, she would give me the injection. So she gave him the prescription, he went down to the pharmacy, got some, and came back. I laid there after the shot. It kind of put my feet to sleep, and I could feel it going up my legs just a little bit at a time, and into my knees, and I thought, "Oh, thank you Lord Jesus. This is going to do something. It's going to get there." By the time it finally got up to where I could feel it a little bit, I could hear that animal sound become quieter. It didn't completely go away, but it was getting more gentle.

DR. KOENIG: Was that all they did? Give you a shot?

PENNY: After a bit, they sat me up, and said, "Okay, well go home and just keep taking the Midrin." And I said, "The Midrin doesn't help me. I'm telling you, I need something else. Just give me something to let me sleep. Just give me something that will take the pain away for just a little while. I can't go on without ammunition again. I just can't take it. Please don't send me home. Put me in the hospital. Watch me. Do something. But don't send me home alone again. I can't take it." At that point, the shot took effect and I was sick as a dog. I relieved myself right there—my bladder went out of control. So that was just lovely. Now I'm humiliated on top of the pain. I'm soaking wet, and my husband's not happy about driving me home in the car. Then I began to vomit. What next?

DR. KOENIG: What kind of a doctor was this?

PENNY: She's either family medicine or internal medicine. When I came home, I told what happened to my next-door neighbor, the family doctor. And she called the doctor who saw me and said, "Listen. I don't usually get involved in these things, and I don't like to, but I need to tell you that you're putting yourself in a bad position suitwise. If she dies of an aneurysm right now, you are going to be in big trouble. She needs some tests done. We need to do something. We need to get some stuff done."

DR. KOENIG: What was the doctor's response to that?

PENNY: At that point, she referred me to a neurologist who had an MRI [magnetic resonance imaging] done, and found out I had some arthritis in my upper lumbar spine or something. But there wasn't anything, no bleed that he could see, and he wanted to put me on Inderal. This time I was ready to take it. I don't know how many days or weeks before the Inderal took effect. I did continue to have migraines after this because Asim took me back in at least on one occasion when I had some kind of IV drip at the hospital. They gave me a steroid drip or something like that, which was supposed to help. And I thought maybe it had helped, and then we got into the car in the parking lot and it started again. So it didn't really help. But after two or three more migraines I finally stopped having them, and, glory to God, I have not had one since.

DR. KOENIG: On the Inderal—the same medication that first neurologist suggested?

PENNY: Yes, Inderal. That's the drug that finally helped me. I'm on Inderal LA, 120 mg tablets, and I take two capsules at bedtime. He had thought I might have some sexual side effects or nightmares, but I did not. I have had no side effects on it. I am also on Depakote, but I don't know if it's helped with my migraines or not.

DR. KOENIG: And how much Depakote are you taking?

PENNY: I lowered myself on the Depakote because I've gained so much weight on it. But I'm taking two tablets, two times a day, and they're 250 mg tablets. I was taking three and three. But I just gained an enormous amount of weight.

DR. KOENIG: Have you ever tried any alternative medical treatments for your headaches?

PENNY: Like acupuncture or something?

DR. KOENIG: Like that, or did you ever take any alternative medicines?

PENNY: No. I didn't know what to take.

DR. KOENIG: You didn't really take anything like that during the nine years of intermittent migraines?

PENNY: Yeah, that's right. Because I was so tough, I just toughed it out.

DR. KOENIG: OK, let's change the subject. How did the pain during that three-week period affect you personally, affect your feelings about yourself?

PENNY: I have to tell you, as it progressed, I became more and more selfish in a way that I'm not proud of. In the beginning I was fighting and I wanted to get better. By the end, I wanted it over so much that I would have rather died than live on in pain. In the beginning, I felt so guilty about poor Asim taking care of everybody and about the kids being without me. By the end I was thinking they'd be better off without me. It really took its toll. I've always prided myself in having such a high pain threshold. But this thing knocked me not only to my knees but down on my face.

DR. KOENIG: How did the pain affect your family life?

PENNY: Everybody felt sorry for me. I'd get occasional visits, but I think they didn't know what to do, and it caused a lot of confusion. I think it was very hard on Asim to go to work every day, and come home and be the wife every night. I think it really did put a strain on us. Asim was not one of these *Little House on the Prairie* husbands who'd say, "I love you, Wife, get better." I felt like he was saying, "Well, if you weren't so fat, this wouldn't have happened to you," or, "Well, if you would just take care of yourself, you wouldn't be in this situation." And I think he sort of blamed me that I hadn't taken better care of myself. If I had, he wouldn't be suffering.

DR. KOENIG: How did the pain affect you spiritually during that time and then afterward?

PENNY: During the time I was in pain, it tested my faith. It truly did because initially I was strong in the Lord. I would think of what Job had gotten through, and I'd know, "Lord, you're going to get me past this." I tried to recite all the Scriptures that I ever knew, so it was kind of good for me. You know, it was good in that way. But as the weeks went on and the pain just continued, like I said, I even tried New Age yoga and meditation practices.

DR. KOENIG: Did that mean you had decided Christianity didn't work?

PENNY: Oh, no, not at all. I never could let go of that. Because I'll tell you the truth, the one thing that Christ gives you is that you might feel helpless, but you never feel hopeless. When I had those negative thoughts, it was during a moment of pure desperation. Do you know what I mean? It would have been one of those just out-of-your-mind-and-not-completely-yourself moments.

DR. KOENIG: But toward the end there—toward the end when you were exhausted and just worn out, you were willing to try anything, right?

PENNY: Yes, I was. But God was still there, you know, I never let Him go. That was my first; when I'd cry, I'd still cry out to Him. And when I'd have any reprieve at all, I would still be praising Him and thanking Him. Since it's been over, the things that I am most thankful for are— you know, it's crazy and it's going to sound weird— but you know how they say there's always a silver lining to every gray cloud? This is a terrible thing that happened to me, and I pray in Jesus' name that I will never ever have one again. I don't know if I could take that. The fear of it is still slightly in me, I hate to say. However, one good thing came out of it.

DR. KOENIG: And what was that?

PENNY: He [God] taught me that my family could in fact get along without me. I mean, I've been such an overfunctioning parent for so long. I've tried to do everything for everybody. When I was in psychotherapy, they asked what I would like to do just for myself. It had been so long since I'd even thought about myself. I had no idea how to respond. I just wanted my children to be happy. I wanted peace in my home. And they said, "No, just for you." I didn't know anything about me. Well, the other week I took a couple of days away with some girlfriends. I never would have done it before that painful time. Asim said, "Go ahead and go." I hadn't asked before because I thought everything would fall apart if I left.

DR. KOENIG: Go on . . .

PENNY: From the three-and-a-half weeks of laying on my back, I learned that everything would not fall apart. The house got a little dirtier, the carpet got dirtier from me not nagging to death, but everyone survived. What it did was knock me down a peg and said, "Penny, dirt is dirt. Life is life. Get on about your business." I think it changed the way I look at life and at my family. I mean, even last night, I had dishes in the sink and laundry to fold, and a neighbor gave us two free tickets to *Lord of the Dance*. And I said, "Is it okay, Asim?" And Tommy and I ran off to *Lord of the Dance*. Dishes are still in the sink. They'll be done tonight. But you know, I would have never done that before. I would have never felt free to do that. So in a way, even though this is a terrible thing that I just keep praying will never happen again, it did change me. I really am thankful for that.

DR. KOENIG: So you do see some value in the pain?

PENNY: There absolutely was value in the pain. I read somewhere that Americans have just gotten so away from pain that we can't take any. And maybe I had been so good at taking pain, I really had to get a good whopping dose before it said, "Hello, Penny."

DR. KOENIG: Can you see any purpose in the pain?

PENNY: Well, if it was God's purpose to open my eyes, then that would certainly be true.

DR. KOENIG: While you were having the pain early on, did you see any purpose for it?

PENNY: It certainly directed my attention to God. I can't tell you since I don't keep a diary, but perhaps I had gotten a little lax in my faith. You know, maybe I had gotten so busy with housework that I wasn't praying as much. That certainly happens in my life a lot. I just get busy and say, "Oh Lord, where have you been the last two months?"

DR. KOENIG: Have you grown as a result of your pain?

PENNY: Yes, I believe that I have grown. Through this, the Lord has taught me more than I know. Even during the time I was saying, "Lord, I don't understand why you're not healing me right now," I knew He was still with me. He said He'd never leave me or forsake me and I knew that He was there, every minute. Even when I was doing the yoga, and focusing on all these different things, I still felt His presence. I did. As I said before, I might have felt helpless, but

I did not feel hopeless. And God did make Himself real to me. Even though I couldn't understand why He was tarrying, why he was waiting so long. My family learned something, and I learned something. He knew what He was doing, and His timing is perfect.

DR. KOENIG: What could your friends or church members have done to help?

PENNY: I would have loved if people had come and prayed with me. I would have loved to have been anointed with oil. But I have to admit, "you have not because you ask not," and I didn't ask a soul. I didn't. How would they have known? I was so sick I couldn't really, and my friends couldn't have gotten here because of the snow anyway. But even with the snow, maybe someone could have prayed with me over the telephone. I think it would have helped me to know that I wasn't alone. You know, sometimes we just need God with skin on.

DR. KOENIG: Is there anything church members or friends really shouldn't do when they're trying to help somebody in pain?

PENNY: Yeah, don't judge somebody at that time. If somebody is in pain, even if it's because she is alcoholic and now she's drying up and having DTs, don't judge her then. Don't say, "Now see what a mess you made? If you didn't make this wrong choice you wouldn't be suffering now." Don't do that. Just say, "Trust in the Lord. Let me pray for you. Is there anything I can do that will make you feel better?" It will turn around later. There are ways to serve others back afterward.

DR. KOENIG: How could your family have helped you—either Asim or the kids?

PENNY: Even though my children, one at a time, came and prayed for me, what a blessing that would have been to have my family gather around me together and pray for me. That would have been such a blessing. I didn't think to ask, but it would have been a real neat thing. I felt kind of abandoned and alone a lot. That was very hard for me during this painful time. There were times when I would have just liked a glass of water. Or I needed a pill and I had to wait. Or I was really hungry and nobody checked on me for the longest period of time. They would finally come, but it just seemed like forever. And I had no bell or calling system or anything. If someone were to check in on the person once an hour to see, do they need something? That would be a good thing.

DR. KOENIG: Last question: What advice would you have for other people who experience pain with headaches?

PENNY: Well, that's tough because I haven't completely solved this yet. I'm still at the point where, if I have another one, I don't even have a pill weapon in my hand. So I still walk around with this tiny seed of fear that it could happen again. I did change doctors. But how do I know if this new doctor is any better? That fear also makes you feel guilty, because the Lord would not want us to have a spirit of fear. I know that. But, in the practical sense, make sure that you take care of yourself, because nobody else is going to take care of you. I hate to have had to learn that lesson. I didn't want to. But I think you have to take care of yourself or find yourself a good doctor that you think knows and understands you. And if that takes shopping around a little to find the right doctor, then do that.

DR. KOENIG: Anything else?

PENNY: Pray a lot. I think you have to pray and confess your fear to the Lord. Just say, "Lord, you know me, every part of me, and my fear as well. I pray for peace and wisdom." And then, you know, certainly read up on the subject. I get this newsletter from a national headache organization now, and it says to avoid chocolate and red wine, and this and that. But there's nothing you can do to avoid the barometric pressure changes that come with the weather, you know. There's all kinds of reasons it happens. So get information, pray, and find a good doctor.

Chapter 5

Rheumatologic Pain—Laura's Story

Laura had been living with chronic pain related to lupus erythematosis for over two decades, first developing symptoms of this autoimmune disease in her mid-twenties. Her mother had the same disease and died from it at an early age. Laura was a patient of mine for nearly ten years. Throughout that time, she dealt with her pain sometimes better, sometimes worse. I'll never forget, however, the visit during the winter when she came in and told me about something her priest had done. On Christmas Day, Laura was unable to attend Mass due to a flare-up of lupus. So her priest came to the hospital and held Mass right at her bedside and administered Holy Communion. This meant so much to her, and she continued to talk about it long afterward.

In the final years, she developed severe right arm pain that was not responsive to any of the treatments offered. During many visits, I would listen to her talk about her pain, helpless to do anything about it. Despite this, I looked forward to those visits because of her great sense of humor. She became severely ill and expired from complications due to lupus about one month after this interview.

DR. KOENIG: When and where were you born?

LAURA: I was born in 1944 in Brooklyn, New York.

DR. KOENIG: What was life like for you as a child?

LAURA: I think it was like any other child growing up in a family that didn't have any money. There was struggling, you know. And my mom was sick so . . . You know what I'm saying?

DR. KOENIG: Your mom had lupus erythematosis, like you, right?

LAURA: Yes, she did. They thought it was rheumatoid arthritis though. It had the same symptoms. I took care of her. And most of the things that have happened to me, I remember, they happened to her. But back then the doctors didn't know much about lupus.

DR. KOENIG: Do you have brothers and sisters?

LAURA: Yes, I have a brother.

DR. KOENIG: How many years of schooling did you complete?

LAURA: All the way up to three years in college.

DR. KOENIG: What kind of job or life aspirations did you have after getting out of school?

LAURA: Well, I didn't have any because my mom was so sick. And I wanted to take care of her and I really didn't have any other desires, you know. I wasn't thinking about anything but taking care of her.

DR. KOENIG: And you did that after you graduated from college?

LAURA: Oh yeah. Uh-huh.

DR. KOENIG: What was the first job that you had?

LAURA: I worked at a telephone company in New York. I started working there I think about 1964, and I worked there until 1975 when we moved to Florida. I got another job for the telephone company and worked there until 1978 when I moved to Durham. Then, I got a job with the phone company there. I worked for about three or four years in Durham, when I had to stop because of my physical condition.

DR. KOENIG: So you stopped work around 1982 because of your condition.

LAURA: I did. I suppose I should have stopped earlier because the doctor told me to think about not working, and I didn't want to think about it because I had my little girl to take care of.

DR. KOENIG: When did you get married?

LAURA: Well, my first husband passed away after seven years of marriage. Until then, we were a normal couple; we lived in New York . . .

DR. KOENIG: What did he die of?

LAURA: Well, somebody killed him.

DR. KOENIG: My, oh, my . . . and then what did you do?

LAURA: Well, just continued to work. I remained single—never remarried.

DR. KOENIG: How old were you when your husband died?

LAURA: I was twenty-six. And now my daughter is already twenty-two.

DR. KOENIG: When did you start experiencing the first symptoms of your condition and the pain?

LAURA: About . . . before she was a year old. I guess because I stopped nursing her. Once I did that, it was just downhill from then on. I got sicker and sicker and sicker and sicker.

DR. KOENIG: What symptoms were you having at that time?

LAURA: Mainly just my legs would hurt. I could hardly walk, and I didn't have any appetite. And—let me see . . . I was so weak. I just didn't have the energy to do anything. And it's been happening on and off since then.

DR. KOENIG: For the past twenty-two years.

LAURA: Yeah, I've been in the hospital lots of times, at least eight times.

DR. KOENIG: Now, let's talk about what limitations your pain causes.

LAURA: Well, it affects my life every day . . . such as taking a shower, even brushing my teeth, because of the movement. And then sometimes it hurts to even brush my hair. I can't do a lot of things that I used to do. I used to go to the YWCA three times a week, and then I couldn't go there anymore. That was something I really liked to do. Then, let's see, it affects most of my daily chores. It's kind of difficult because it takes me longer to do things than it used to. I do them, but I have to struggle.

DR. KOENIG: What things, for example, do you struggle with, that most people do without thinking?

LAURA: I struggle with walking up the stairs. I struggle with getting my pants on. I struggle with buttoning them up. You know buttons? I don't do buttons at all. And, well, I struggle with walking. And washing dishes. I struggle with holding a glass in my left hand. I always waste everything I do with my left arm because I don't have the strength to hold things in that hand.

DR. KOENIG: Describe your pain. What is your pain like?

LAURA: It's actually all over. But mostly—what really gets my attention a whole lot—is the pain in my arm. What is it like? Well, let's see. If you were to have electricity running up and down your arm, you know. . . . like little, I don't know what you'd call them . . .

DR. KOENIG: Shocks?

LAURA: Little shocks going up and down the arm, that's right. And then sometimes just outright pain to the touch.

DR. KOENIG: Even just to the touch?

LAURA: Just to the touch, really. Because my body is so sore. And I don't know why that is.

DR. KOENIG: Is it that way throughout the day?

LAURA: Throughout the day. Uh-huh.

DR. KOENIG: What about at night?

LAURA: Oh, at night it just gets worse. Mainly I sit up. I have a kind of chair that gives you a massage. I sleep in that most of the time.

DR. KOENIG: You don't lie down?

LAURA: No, because I have trouble breathing, so I don't lie down a lot. I usually sleep sitting up.

DR. KOENIG: How many hours of good sleep do you get a night?

LAURA: I don't know. I'm always up and down, up and down, up and down. I'd say maybe about a good hour without getting up. I get up and lay back down, and then I have to get up again, you know . . .

DR. KOENIG: Why are you so restless at night?

LAURA: I really don't know.

DR. KOENIG: Is it the pain, or is it just . . . ?

LAURA: The pain is the main thing, actually.

DR. KOENIG: Is your pain there when you wake up in the morning?

LAURA: Yes.

DR. KOENIG: And when you go to bed at night?

LAURA: Yes.

DR. KOENIG: Does it ever go away?

LAURA: No, I've actually learned to live with it. I know that I'm going to be hurting. And I know that this is going to be happening to me all day so I just try to live with it. It's better on the days that I rest. Then one day I get up and I say, "Oh jeez, no pain. I feel pretty good." Then I overexert myself and the pain comes back.

DR. KOENIG: How often do you wake up without pain?

LAURA: Not often. Pain free? Very, very seldom.

DR. KOENIG: How many times in a month does that happen?

LAURA: Oh . . . maybe once a week, maybe.

DR. KOENIG: Have pain medications helped?

LAURA: Yeah, the medications have actually helped my pain a whole lot. Before I was taking the medications, I mean I was just in constant pain all the time . . . it never let up.

DR. KOENIG: What medicine really helps?

LAURA: Well, let's see, the Percocet helps.

DR. KOENIG: How much time does it take before the pain starts to ease up?

LAURA: It starts easing off a little bit after about forty-five minutes. Then I feel the medicine getting into my system, and I'm not hurting as bad.

DR. KOENIG: And how long does the relief last?

LAURA: Well, actually, it lasts about three hours maybe.

DR. KOENIG: Are you pain free during that time?

LAURA: No.

DR. KOENIG: You still have pain.

LAURA: Yes. And I know toward the end of that three hours that pretty soon I'm going to have to take a pain pill. Otherwise, I feel like jumping out the window. It makes you nervous. It makes you jittery all the time.

DR. KOENIG: The pain does?

LAURA: Yeah, you're always jittery.

DR. KOENIG: Have you ever had surgery for your pain?

LAURA: No, I haven't.

DR. KOENIG: Have you tried any alternative medicines, natural or organic substances, or nontraditional treatments to ease your pain?

LAURA: I've tried stuff at the Wellspring store (organic food store). [Bob also tried medicines he bought at the Wellspring store.]

DR. KOENIG: What kinds of alternative medicines have you tried?

LAURA: I can't even think of the name of the pills. One was something to help me sleep.

DR. KOENIG: Some natural substance?

LAURA: Yeah. I can't even remember what it was. It was a long time ago.

DR. KOENIG: Did that help much?

LAURA: No.

DR. KOENIG: What else? Anything else? For the pain in particular.

LAURA: They had some stuff that you rub on your arms, but it didn't help. It just burned. It just burned a whole lot and it smelled icky, but it didn't help a bit.

DR. KOENIG: Can you think of anything else you may have tried that was natural or organic, something that people claim helps pain?

LAURA: Well, I went to the Duke pain clinic. I could tell you about that.

DR. KOENIG: Did the pain clinic help?

LAURA: No.

DR. KOENIG: What did they do there?

LAURA: Well, you have to listen to these tapes, and think of all kinds of things that are supposed to make you feel better.

DR. KOENIG: You mean like relaxation?

LAURA: Right.

DR. KOENIG: And imagery?

LAURA: You're right. Imagine that you are at a beach, and it's warm. But they tried this approach with me in the dead of winter, so, you know, it's not that warm. The winter is when my Raynaud's really starts giving me a lot of trouble. [Raynaud's is a condition associated with lupus erythematosis in which the blood vessels in the hands and feet constrict in response to cold, causing severe pain.] They were trying to help me so I could walk, and do something so my hands wouldn't turn blue.

DR. KOENIG: What else did they do? Did you try anything else? Biofeedback or . . . ?

LAURA: Oh yeah, I tried that, biofeedback. And groups.

DR. KOENIG: They had groups for pain?

LAURA: Yeah, they had groups for pain.

DR. KOENIG: Did that help?

LAURA: Nope. It is fine to sit around and talk, but it wasn't helping me. I mean I wasn't getting any benefit out of it so I was wasting time when I could be laying down, taking a nap (if I could), or just being absolutely quiet.

DR. KOENIG: How has the pain affected you personally—how you feel about yourself?

LAURA: It makes you depressed. Say you want to go out, get all dressed up, but you can't do it because of the pain.

DR. KOENIG: What about how you feel about yourself? You know, your self-image. Does the pain affect that?

LAURA: Yeah. You walk around having the blahs all the time and you feel like everybody says, "Well, you're bugging me, I can't do this for you, and I don't have time to do that for you." I feel like I'm a burden to other people, weighing people down.

DR. KOENIG: And that doesn't make you feel very good.

LAURA: No, because I don't want to be, you know, a burden. But I can still drive, thank the Lord. And that means I can go anyplace I want to go. But I don't have the strength to go.

DR. KOENIG: Do you feel tired a lot?

LAURA: Oh yeah, that's what I've been having lately, more and more fatigue. And the doctor increased my folic acid pills but that didn't help a bit. We thought it was going to help, but it didn't. He went down on my methotrexate pills, just in one week he went down by two pills. I was taking six every Friday, but he said well, we'll just take four. That week that I took four pills I had the worst pain in my arm that I've ever had. But he said it didn't have anything to do with the methotrexate because it wouldn't have gotten out of my system that fast. But since I had been on it a long time, and I felt it had already kicked in. So if you mess with the dose, you're going to feel it.

DR. KOENIG: That makes sense. Are you taking steroids too?

LAURA: Yeah.

DR. KOENIG: Prednisone?

LAURA: Yeah.

DR. KOENIG: How much of that do you take?

LAURA: Well right now I'm on forty milligrams per day. I've got the sores in my mouth from the lupus. They're trying to clear those up, but it's not working. Yesterday, I got up, and my mouth wasn't hurting. I was surprised; I said, "Oh geez, it's over." Then after I got up and brushed my teeth, it was right back.

DR. KOENIG: Let me switch topics now. How has the pain affected your relationships with your relatives, with your daughter, with other members of your family?

LAURA: It really hasn't affected them too bad.

DR. KOENIG: It hasn't?

LAURA: No, because I don't complain to them, you know. I don't go, "Oh, I'm so sick." Doing that makes me feel worse. So, I don't complain to them. I just try to go on and act just like I normally would act.

DR. KOENIG: What about doing things with your daughter?

LAURA: Every Saturday we go shopping.

DR. KOENIG: Does your physical pain ever limit your ability to do stuff with your daughter?

LAURA: Oh yeah.

DR. KOENIG: For example, how does the pain affect it?

LAURA: For example, when it gets hot outside [in July], like you know, between 10:00 a.m. and 4:00 p.m., I can barely breathe outside. It's so hot, it burns me. So I try not to go out during those hours. But sometimes I'm caught out there, and my body realizes I shouldn't be out there, and it starts aching. And air conditioning is not for me. I feel sometimes like I could just be hot and forget the air conditioning. But you can't because otherwise you can't breathe.

DR. KOENIG: How has your pain affected you spiritually?

LAURA: Well, I go to church a lot more. I go to Mass a lot more than I used to.

DR. KOENIG: And why do you do that?

LAURA: I go to pray. You know, just talk to the Lord and get some complete quietness. And pray that I'll get along today, that today will be a better day than yesterday, that my spirits will be higher than yesterday. That really breaks you down a lot.

DR. KOENIG: What does?

LAURA: When you complain about . . . "Oh, I'm so sick." And you feel like you want to cry because you're hurting so bad. That breaks you down a whole lot.

DR. KOENIG: And how does your spirituality influence that?

LAURA: I just start saying my prayers.

DR. KOENIG: Does that help?

LAURA: Actually, yes.

DR. KOENIG: What does it do for you?

LAURA: It makes me feel good. I'll put it to you like this. I feel better about myself when I go to church. That's the only place that I feel complete. I mean, I just feel good about myself in church. But the key is, I'm so thankful that I can still go. Because if you don't have nobody to take you, you can't go. And in the wintertime I can't see at night so good. I can't see to drive. So I have to be taken during the winter. But now since it's light a long time, I can still go.

DR. KOENIG: What about when you're at home? Do you do anything at home, spiritually, that lifts you up?

LAURA: Oh yeah, I say my prayers, and say my Rosary, and I'll read the Bible a little, read a part of the Scripture.

DR. KOENIG: You do those things because they do what?

LAURA: They make me feel uplifted. They uplift me.

DR. KOENIG: What kinds of questions do you ask God?

LAURA: I've never asked him why, because he knows why.

DR. KOENIG: Did you ever in the past ask God why?

LAURA: No, because he knows why. I've gotten to the point where I know it's going to be this way. This is the way it's going to be, you know. Go on and do the best you can, and what you can't do, you can't do. What you can do, you do.

DR. KOENIG: So you haven't asked God why?

LAURA: No, because I feel like God doesn't put any more on you than you can bear. Like if you were going to have a baby, and the baby was sick. I don't think he would give a sick baby to somebody who couldn't handle it. Me, myself, I don't think I could handle a sick baby. I didn't have a sick baby. Oh, that would just tear me up. And the people that do have the babies that are sick seem to handle it very well. But I couldn't.

DR. KOENIG: Do you ask God any other questions?

LAURA: Oh yeah. I sometimes ask him that if I'm not going to have any more mobility, if I'm not going to feel any better than this, if I can't eat without hurting—I just don't want to be here. And then something comes into my mind: "Don't say that, because you do want to be here." Because you don't know about the hereafter. It may be worse than here, who knows. We don't know.

DR. KOENIG: What could your friends, church members, do to help you with your pain?

LAURA: I guess, stick with me when I'm down. And understanding when I just don't feel well at all. And my friends know that about me. They know exactly when I don't feel well. They can hear it in my voice.

DR. KOENIG: What do they do for you when they sense that?

LAURA: Well, they don't do anything that really, really helps, but we try to talk. And we try to, you know, plan on going out to dinner, and stuff like that. Just to get my mind off of being sick. Because they know that there's really nothing they can do. But anything that they could, they would. I know that.

DR. KOENIG: Are your friends mostly in your church, or are they outside of your church?

LAURA: Well, most of my friends when I was working were outside of the church. And now, most of my friends are from my church. And then, you know, my daughter's friend's parents, you know, I met them through her activities. [pause] I used to pray when I first started getting sick. I used to ask God, "Just let me live long enough for my daughter to be able to take care of herself." So I wouldn't have to worry about her being taken care of. She's able to take care of herself now, and if I pass away, then it won't be so bad on her. She knows how to take care of herself now.

DR. KOENIG: What do friends or church members do that really does *not* help?

LAURA: When they just go overboard to do these things that they think would make me happy, you know, and make me feel better. Sometimes they write me notes. That's fine. But sometimes I don't even feel like reading. But they don't understand that, so I don't say anything to them. I just thank them and I go on. And then I have friends that, they get a headache, and they're crying all the time. And that makes me upset. I say, if you could just walk one day in my shoes, you wouldn't be doing this much crying. You wouldn't be hurting as bad. [Remember Bob's words: almost the same idea expressed.]

I've got a friend like that right now. She has fibromyalgia, and it's just killing her. . . . She just can't stand any kind of pain, period. Every little thing tears her up. So you know how she's doing; she's not doing well at all. And then I feel guilty when she comes to pick me up on Saturday to go to church, because she doesn't feel good. I mean, I know she doesn't feel good, because she cries all the time.

DR. KOENIG: And so that makes you feel guilty?

LAURA: Yeah, for having to ride with her.

DR. KOENIG: That she has to pick you up?

LAURA: Yeah. Some of the time she doesn't have to pick me up, but she still picks me up anyway. We still go to church together. At least she really cares. You know, there are a lot of people in church that say they care about you, but they really don't. They put on a big show.

DR. KOENIG: Tell me about that.

LAURA: You know, like there's one lady in particular that tries to pretend. She says, "I just don't know how you do it. I just don't know how you get around." I say, "I get around." She says, "I just don't understand it." I say, "There's nothing here to understand." And then she'll say, "Well, I'll come over, and I'll help you do a few things around the house." But she's not coming. And she's going to say this in a group of people so they can hear her saying it, and so she can hear herself say it, but she's not going to come.

DR. KOENIG: So, it's all superficial.

LAURA: Like I said, the only friend that I really and truly can say I have is the one that takes me back and forth to church. I met her at work. She's from Connecticut. And she's been my friend ever since I've been back here.

DR. KOENIG: Is that the one with fibromyalgia?

LAURA: Yeah, that's the one. And she just cries all the time in church. I just feel so sorry for her; I don't know what to do.

DR. KOENIG: What could your family do to help you with your pain? What could your daughter do? That's your main family, right?

LAURA: Yeah.

DR. KOENIG: What could she do to help you with your pain?

LAURA: I think maybe coming over, coming by to see me. I get a lot of joy out of that. She's so excited now about her new job, she loves it, and she's telling me about all the people at work there, and all the things that they do. You know, I just kind of get involved in her work. But one thing I do miss, I miss reading. I can't concentrate long enough to read, because the pain makes me stop. I just hate that. Even most of the prayers that I say, they are very short.

DR. KOENIG: Would it help if your daughter read to you?

LAURA: No, I want to read to myself. And not aloud. I wouldn't want . . . Oh, I don't know . . . I just don't want to be a burden to any-body. That's the main thing.

DR. KOENIG: What if your daughter wanted to help you with your pain? What could she do? She comes by and visits you and that gives you joy; what else?

LAURA: Well, if there's something that needs to be done around the house, and I'm not able to do it, she'll go do it for me. That's a joy, because if I can't do it, I've got to have somebody to do it. Just sim-ple things, that, you know, anybody could do, open a jar . . . I can't do that. But she'll do things like that. Fix my bed, and help me get in and out of the tub, and things like that.

DR. KOENIG: If you could tell your daughter or other family members what they should *not* do for someone struggling with pain, what would you say?

LAURA: Don't complain to me. Please don't.

DR. KOENIG: Don't complain about pain to you?

LAURA: No, no, I don't want that at all.

DR. KOENIG: Anything else?

LAURA: Don't tell me, "I know how you feel," because you don't know how I feel. Nobody could know how you feel—not unless they were you. They would have to be you to really know.

DR. KOENIG: What has helped you the most in coping with your pain?

LAURA: Praying. Praying has helped me more than anything. And when I'm home alone, that helps a lot. That's the main thing. And I know that if I say my prayers, it's all going to be okay.

DR. KOENIG: Can you tell a difference in the level of pain?

LAURA: Yeah, it goes down. Because I think it gives me something else to think about. It's frustrating because you think about what you used to do, and now what you can't do. It's really frustrating. It's depressing when you do that. But prayer helps.

DR. KOENIG: Can you see any value in your pain? Is there anything good in your pain?

LAURA: Good? No.

DR. KOENIG: Do you see any value in the pain?

LAURA: Well, I can help other people. I listen to them. Even though they know I don't like them to complain. And they say, after they're finished, "I shouldn't have said that to you." But I listen.

DR. KOENIG: And so, your ability to listen, is that something good that has resulted from your pain?

LAURA: Well, yeah.

DR. KOENIG: Tell me about that.

LAURA: I can concentrate on them and not concentrate on myself. I have something else to think about.

DR. KOENIG: What you're saying is that if there's any good in your pain, it helps you listen to others?

LAURA: Oh yes. And understand.

DR. KOENIG: You understand what they're going through.

LAURA: Uh-huh, because sometimes they don't understand what they're going through. And they're always saying, "Why me?" and all that. You don't know why. The Lord picks you for this because you can take it. He doesn't give you more than you can handle.

DR. KOENIG: The good in your pain is that it gives you understanding?

LAURA: Yes it does. Of other people. And keeps me from focusing on myself. And when I do that, I don't feel as bad.

DR. KOENIG: Have you ever thought, "What purpose could this pain have?"

LAURA: No, I never really thought about it like that. I say, you know, this is just the way it's going to be. There's nothing I can do about it. No, there's no purpose in this.

DR. KOENIG: Then why would a loving God enable you to have it?

LAURA: Because he knows that I can take it.

DR. KOENIG: But why would he allow you to go through it?

LAURA: Because he knows that I'm strong enough to take it. Mentally. Maybe not physically, sometimes, but mentally I can take it. And that makes me really have sympathy for others that are in pain. When I know that they can't take things. A little bit of pain just knocks them out and they're dead. So I just feel sorry for them because they just can't focus on, you know, the pretty flowers. You know. The sun outside. And being able to just walk outside.

DR. KOENIG: So it gives you sympathy for those people.

LAURA: Yes, it does. It really does.

DR. KOENIG: So, in that sense it maybe does give you something?

LAURA: Yeah, it does. It gives me that.

DR. KOENIG: How have you grown as a result of your pain?

LAURA: Well, I try to help others. I try to be a caregiver, which I am, really. I'm a caregiver. And I've always been that way.

DR. KOENIG: Has your pain helped you be that way more?

LAURA: Yes. Because some of the things that I can do, I do them for other people. Like I go and help serve the homeless. We go over there once a month and give them a dinner. And I go help them do that. I can barely pick up the spoon, it's so heavy, but I just go on and do the best that I can. And when it gets to the point where I just can't lift it anymore, I just stop. And everybody understands why I stop. But I try, and I try to make something to take . . . something that you can just put in the oven.

DR. KOENIG: You help out at the homeless shelter.

LAURA: Yeah. We go there once a month, and give them a nice dinner, a lovely dinner really. And they enjoy it. They love it. It's so . . . it's homemade, somebody's standing there dishing it out to you. . . . The only thing you've got to do is stand there and hold your plate. That's all you've got to do.

DR. KOENIG: Here is the final question. What kind of advice would you have for other people like yourself with chronic pain? How would you advise them?

LAURA: Get pain medication, and learn how to control it. You know, they say you can take one pill every four hours. Learn how to not take that extra one . . . just take that one, and let it go. Just hurt a little bit, but not too much. You don't want to be too uncomfortable. Just make the pain so you can deal with it.

DR. KOENIG: So, take pain medication. . . . What else?

LAURA: Get a good rest in the afternoon. Don't get up early if you don't feel good. And don't do things that you know are going to hurt you later. I can say, "Oh, I feel so good. I feel much better than I've felt in a long time. Let me do some of this. Let me do that." That's the worst thing to do. Don't do it.

DR. KOENIG: What about coping with the pain? What advice would you give?

LAURA: Don't let pain be your whole focus in life. If that's your whole focus, you're not going to be in this world for much longer. You're going to worry yourself to death. That's the main thing— don't let it be your whole focus. Focus on something else.

DR. KOENIG: Any other advice?

LAURA: Focus on things that you can do something about. Don't focus on the things you can't do anything about. If you do, you're going to be miserable.

DR. KOENIG: Don't focus on things you can't control.

LAURA: Right, because you're going to be miserable if you do. That's the main thing. And don't focus on yourself. Because you'll be crying all the time . . . and you'll be feeling sorry for yourself. Don't focus on yourself.

Chapter 6

Generalized Pain—Jackie's Story

I have known Jackie for nearly ten years. She lives with her husband, and they have a counseling ministry. She has struggled with chronic pain throughout most of the time I've known her, despite multiple surgeries and high doses of narcotic pain relievers to control the pain. Through it all, she has maintained a very strong spirit, and there is a special quality about the way she bears her pain. Jackie is known throughout her church community as a "prayer warrior," and those who are suffering gravitate to her like iron to a magnet. Always ready to encourage, always ready to support, always ready to give hope and prayer—that's Jackie—even when she's having pain.

DR. KOENIG: When were you born and where?

JACKIE: I was born October 23, 1949, in a small town in West Virginia.

DR. KOENIG: Tell me what it was like growing up.

JACKIE: My grandfather and grandmother were retired and they had a farm. I grew up on a farm next to their property. And so we had horses and an apple orchard and a garden and all kinds of things like that.

DR. KOENIG: How many siblings did you have?

JACKIE: One brother and one sister.

DR. KOENIG: Were those early years difficult?

JACKIE: Not until I was eight, I guess, when my father began to get sick. He was vice president of a natural gas company. He traveled all week long in the northeastern part of the United States, coming home only on weekends. But then he began to get sick, which resulted in us having to suddenly move. He'd been to the Mayo

Clinic, Johns Hopkins, the Cleveland Clinic, and some clinic in Pittsburgh. They all said that he had to move to a climate that would be better for his health and gave him two choices. One was Arizona and the other was Florida.

DR. KOENIG: What kind of health condition did he have?

JACKIE: He had a bleeding ulcer and a gallbladder that ruptured at the same time, requiring the removal of about ninety-three percent of his stomach. Then he also had different types of arthritis, two different types of arthritis that I remember, and some other bone and joint problems. So he could not endure the kind of climate where it was cold in the winter.

DR. KOENIG: Did he live very long after that?

JACKIE: Yes, he lived to be eighty-three years old. He outlived my mother.

DR. KOENIG: How old was he when you were ten years old?

JACKIE: He was in his forties. He was forced to retire from his job when that happened. And we were plucked up out of the farm environment in the country and moved to Fort Lauderdale, Florida, which was obviously totally different. Going into junior high school at age eleven, I guess, was like going from bobby socks to panty hose overnight. It was a shock, a real shock for everybody. I never wanted to leave West Virginia. I spent more time at my grandmother's than I did at home, so I had a real attachment to her. She was more like a mother to me in many ways than a grandmother.

DR. KOENIG: How many years of schooling did you finish, and what kind of life aspirations did you have after getting out of school?

JACKIE: I went to four years of college and got my degree. When I got out of high school, I was confused. My grades weren't good enough to go to nursing school, or physical therapy, or something in that field. I didn't really have a direction. So I got a business degree, although I didn't really know what to do with it. I started working during high school in sales and retail. I ended up working twenty-five years in retail in one form or another. I worked for Jordan Marsh's department store and got trained as a buyer, and then went to work for another company.

DR. KOENIG: So you worked as a retailer.

JACKIE: Women's clothing, primarily.

DR. KOENIG: For twenty-five years?

JACKIE: Well, yes, on and off. But not just in women's clothing, although it was the primary focus. I've worked as a bridal consultant, where I sold bridal gowns and organized weddings. I worked as a florist for awhile. I worked as a manager of a jewelry store. But it was all retail, different aspects of retail.

DR. KOENIG: When did you last work?

JACKIE: The last part-time job I had was in 1996, I suppose, and the last full-time job was in 1989.

DR. KOENIG: When did you get married, and how did you meet your husband, Steve?

JACKIE: It's a long story. We got married in 1989. It may sound strange, but I knew I was going to marry him in 1984. I saw him and I knew I was going to marry him. We were at a church conference in Dallas, Texas. There were about five thousand people. He didn't know me, and I didn't know him. I knew who he was, but that was all. I'd never met him.

DR. KOENIG: How did you know of him?

JACKIE: I was in his son Billy's church when it first started, when Billy and Louanne had only been married two weeks. That was in 1982. Steve lived in California and I lived here in Durham, North Carolina. He was in a church in California, but he was at the church conference when I first saw him in 1984. He was sitting with Billy and Louanne. I still didn't meet him at that time. I just knew I was going to marry him. And I began to pray for him. I didn't really know exactly what I was praying for, but I began to pray for him anyway. The Lord just kept reassuring me that he would live here in Durham someday and the whole thing was going to work out. In 1988, he moved to Durham, we met formally and after a brief courtship got married.

DR. KOENIG: Was that your first marriage?

JACKIE: No, my second.

DR. KOENIG: When and how long were you married the first time?

JACKIE: In 1970 I married my first husband, and that lasted for about ten years. It should have never been. People get married for different reasons. We both wanted to be out of our family situations and thought it might be a good idea.

DR. KOENIG: Did you have any kids with that marriage?

JACKIE: No. I lost one. I had one child and lost it.

DR. KOENIG: During the pregnancy?

JACKIE: No. The child died at the age of about seven weeks. That was in 1973.

DR. KOENIG: I'm sorry. That must have been a rough experience.

JACKIE: Yes, it was.

DR. KOENIG: Tell me how and when your physical pain started.

JACKIE: I had several problems with my uterus. I had a terrible time with my menstrual cycle from the very beginning. But it was after about 1972 I kept having painful cysts, you know, that would rupture. And the doctors did a couple of minor surgeries. Anyway, it developed into endometriosis and it got so bad that I had to have a hysterectomy in 1979.

DR. KOENIG: And did that help with the pain?

JACKIE: With that particular pain, yes. But the repercussions of it . . . I planned on having a vaginal hysterectomy, but when I woke up I learned I'd had a total hysterectomy. I was twenty-nine years old, and could never have any more children. I had the onset of menopausal symptoms immediately, even while I was in the hospital. Then they put me on all kinds of hormones to try to counteract the emotional upset. I was soaking wet almost all the time. I couldn't function or think very well. It was pretty traumatic. At that point in time, they didn't have anything except progesterone and Provera, so I got blood clots in both legs. I was hospitalized about five times in six months for that.

DR. KOENIG: How did the pain gradually become chronic?

JACKIE: Even before then there were several instances where I had pain in one leg. I was athletic during my teenage years. I was a swimmer. I was used to having pulled muscles. But one time in my twenties I remember my leg just gave out, and so they sent me to a neurologist. It happened again right at the beginning of my thirties, where both my leg and arm gave out. The muscles just went lax. And then I had this sharp pain up my back. Both of those times, the neurologist asked me if anybody in my family had ever had multiple sclerosis. I said no, not to my knowledge, so they never explored it any further. These bouts began to develop into chronic pain. Also around 1979 I was involved in two car accidents. I was separated from my first husband and going through a divorce. The car accidents caused a lot of injuries, which led from one surgery to another. Both times I was hit by a drunk driver.

DR. KOENIG: That has caused recurrent, ongoing pain for the last twenty years?

JACKIE: Yes, and several surgeries.

DR. KOENIG: What kind of limitations does your pain cause now?

JACKIE: Well, there are some days that I can't feel my hand or my arm, but I can feel this pain in the back of my neck. I can't lift my arm up to comb my hair or brush my teeth with my right hand. There are some days that I have to limp, so I use a cane. There are some days I can't sit for more than fifteen minutes at a time. There are some days I can't drive my car. There are some nights I don't sleep at all. I mean some nights, not every night. The pain is always there, but the intensity of it sometimes increases to an intolerable level.

DR. KOENIG: Where is the pain located?

JACKIE: Most of it is on my right side. Some of it is on my left side. At this point in time there are several types of pain going on. The main pain that is debilitating is the nerve pain that I feel in my face, my right arm, my right shoulder, and the chest wall on my right side.

DR. KOENIG: What is that pain like?

JACKIE: Most of the time it's a burning pain. If it starts in one place like my arm or shoulder, and if I don't get control of the pain, it ends up extending into the back of my head. This pain feels like an electric jolt and stops me dead in my tracks. It completely immobilizes me. I have to learn other ways to do things in order to maintain some sort of normalcy in my life. The other kind of pain I have is bone and joint pain. And it feels anywhere from numbing to aching to squeezing. It feels so deep that you couldn't get to it if you had to rub it, or if somebody else tried to rub it. I don't know a lot of people with that kind of pain.

DR. KOENIG: Give me an example of a typical day.

JACKIE: On most days, I wake up with pain. And then it all depends on what I do that day. Most days the pain is there. I might have two or three days where the intensity eases off some. Last week we went away on vacation for three days. It was always there. The whole first day it was there. But the rest of the time, all we did was walk on the beach, go out to eat, stay at home and read, that kind of thing. As long as I wasn't moving for very long, it was fine. But of course it's made worse by the heat—more so the humidity than the heat.

DR. KOENIG: And activity makes it worse?

JACKIE: Sometimes it does. I guess there's no real pattern to it, but activity generally makes it worse. Sometimes I can do absolutely nothing and yet the pain becomes so extreme, it's just ridiculous.

DR. KOENIG: What about toward evening time?

JACKIE: Usually by 8:30 or 9:00 p.m., at least during the week, it's time to slow down. Work's over, and I can relax. I have to lie down in a chair where I can lift my legs up.

DR. KOENIG: And then the pain gets better?

JACKIE: Well, at least it's tolerable. I usually have to take some kind of pain medication at that time. I've found that even the weakest kind of pain medication that I take during the day affects my mind and makes it clouded. In my work as a counselor, I can't sit through a session if I can't function. When I'm involved in something spiritual, like during counseling, it's almost like I can shut myself off from the pain. At those times, when I'm having pain, that's when the Lord uses me the most to help people. And I have no idea why that is, other than that He says in our weakness, He'll be made strong.

DR. KOENIG: We're going to talk about that in a minute. What about at night? Does the pain keep you from sleeping soundly?

JACKIE: Yes, it wakes me up. I go to bed anywhere from 9:30 to 10:00 p.m. and I'll sleep pretty well until maybe 1:30 a.m., and then I get up for awhile. Then I might go back to sleep for an hour, but I'm up every hour or hour and a half through the rest of the night because of the pain.

DR. KOENIG: Have medications helped your pain?

JACKIE: Sometimes, in the short term.

DR. KOENIG: What kinds of medicines seem to help?

JACKIE: Primarily, narcotic painkillers like Locet and Oxycontin.

DR. KOENIG: Do anti-inflammatory drugs like ibuprofen or medicine like Tylenol help much?

JACKIE: No, they don't.

DR. KOENIG: Do they help at all?

JACKIE: Only sometimes, when there's some inflammation or swelling going on.

DR. KOENIG: Any other medicines?

JACKIE: I've taken steroid pills, but they're short term. The ones I have a problem with are the medications that fog my mind. So before I take them, I have to figure out what the trade-off is going to be, particularly if I'm counseling that day.

DR. KOENIG: Has surgery helped ease your pain?

JACKIE: Yes, some of them have.

DR. KOENIG: What kinds of surgeries have you had in the past ten years?

JACKIE: I've had three back surgeries. The last one was the most severe.

DR. KOENIG: When did you have that one?

JACKIE: About two years ago.

DR. KOENIG: Did it help?

JACKIE: Yes, I think the last one has helped.

DR. KOENIG: Have any alternative medical treatments or natural substances helped your pain?

JACKIE: I don't think so, although they may have helped the course of the disease. I think vitamins and other organic things naturally help your health. Physical therapy has helped, at least in the short term.

DR. KOENIG: How has the pain affected you personally and your feelings about yourself?

JACKIE: If I allowed myself the privilege of feeling sorry for myself, then it might affect me. But I don't do that.

DR. KOENIG: What if you did?

JACKIE: I would probably be very depressed and withdrawn. This feeling that nobody understands. I don't think it would offer me much hope.

DR. KOENIG: How has your pain affected your relationship with your husband?

JACKIE: It's probably enhanced our relationship through the many trials it has put us through. It's given me a greater sense of compassion for him and for what he has to go through to put up with me sometimes. A lot of times the pain has control of me, before I recognize what is going on. He can recognize it quicker than I can.

DR. KOENIG: Has the pain affected your relationship with your husband in a negative way?

JACKIE: Nothing more than that it prevents us from being as spontaneous, probably, as we'd like to be with our life. It's caused me to have to make different kinds of plans for things that normally would just be taken care of. For example, our business is in our home. So every day our home has to look like we're going to have visitors. So pushing the vacuum cleaner, dusting—all those things have to be done before somebody walks in here early in the morning. And if I can't do it, I have to make arrangements with my husband so that he can. So, you know, you just have to make different plans for life.

DR. KOENIG: How has your pain affected you spiritually?

JACKIE: It's given me the ability, not only the ability but the desire, to see God in a different way than I would if the pain wasn't there.

DR. KOENIG: Tell me more about that.

JACKIE: In the Bible, it talks about how He understands everything that we go through, that He was tempted by everything. So He understands everything about my pain. He understands on the days that I hate it. He understands on the days that I don't understand it. And yet at the same time, He's not going anywhere. He's still there for me, and I'm still there for Him. It's made me recognize that it's not all about me; it's about Him.

DR. KOENIG: What else?

JACKIE: It's made me much more aware of the people around me and their problems, and the depth of those problems, and the pain in those problems. Why? I can identify with that pain to a degree that

I'm sure I couldn't if I didn't have pain myself. It's given me a greater ability to be patient. I'm not saying I'm always patient, because I'm not. But it's helped me to be kinder, more tolerant of other people and their situations. I understand their pain.

DR. KOENIG: What kinds of questions do you ask God?

JACKIE: What purpose is being served out of the pain, and how can He use it? I used to ask if it was ever going to be over. I didn't get an answer, so I don't know about that. People tell me, though, that He does use my pain to help others. I don't understand how He uses it. I know how I feel on the inside. I feel like He's . . . There's a scripture in Colossians 1:24 that talks about entering into the sufferings of Christ. It's specifically about Paul preaching the Gospel, and how he takes on the sufferings of Christ for those around him. Not that Christ didn't, you know, take everything for all of us on the cross. Paul wasn't dismissing what Christ did in any way, but it's the closest thing that I can come to understanding what taking on the sufferings of other people involves. Sometimes not in martyrdom, but in love, to see that they're built up and released into whatever God has for them.

DR. KOENIG: Go on.

JACKIE: I'm also interested in prayer, and I believe I have a gift of intercession. So it seems like during the times of greatest pain, that's when God uses me—through intercession in prayer—to help others the most. And then somewhere down the road, I'll see it—the fruit of the intercession.

DR. KOENIG: Anything else?

JACKIE: I can always go to Him when the pain is intolerable.

DR. KOENIG: Is God the only person that you can go to?

JACKIE: Well, I can go to my husband, but he's not going to understand like God is. I can't expect him to. I can't expect anybody to. I've come to that realization. I've come to the conclusion that there are some times that people just don't understand those things.

DR. KOENIG: Do you ever get angry at God over the pain?

JACKIE: I'm not sure I get angry at Him. I get angry at the pain, on occasion. It gets to be more than I can bear, or more than I think that I can bear sometimes. No, I used to get angry at God, but I don't think I do anymore.

DR. KOENIG: Used to get angry? Until when?

JACKIE: I don't know. Probably a year ago. The anger began to ease up, and I finally began to see . . . that God was using me through this pain.

DR. KOENIG: What can your friends or members of your church do to help you with your pain?

JACKIE: There's a lot of people that pray for me and that helps. That's probably the greatest help. On occasion it helps to have somebody you can just vent your frustration to or simply talk to. You don't want them to fix you. You just want to talk to them about it, just get it out.

DR. KOENIG: What do you mean?

JACKIE: People are uncomfortable when you have problems, especially if you're viewed as a strong person. It makes them uncomfortable when you talk about your pain, and they want to come to your aid in some way. This is the answer or that is the answer . . . but there is no answer. So I don't talk about it with many people. If people ask me how I'm doing at church, I'll just ask them to pray for me. But I don't go into any great depth with very many people. Because a lot of times I've found that if they don't have an answer, or they can't find an answer, and you keep describing it, they start feeling sorry for you, and then their misery becomes your misery. That is not helpful; it's not healing. The only thing that kind of sympathy does is make you go deeper down, instead of lifting you up. So if you can be lifted up to God by somebody's prayers, I say that's the greatest help.

DR. KOENIG: What else?

JACKIE: Of course, there's also practical help, you know, on days that you can't do certain things, I mean I'll have people make meals for me, or, you know, I have a friend who comes once in awhile and cleans my house, or helps me clean this or that if I can't do it.

DR. KOENIG: So church members and friends can help you by listening to you, praying for you, and doing practical things for you around the house.

JACKIE: They should first find out what the person's needs are. They should find out really what the needs are, not through another person, but directly from the person in pain. A lot of people tend to be intimidated by the pain. For example, they might say, "Oh, I'll pray for her," or "Oh, well how can I pray for you?" It just comes across trite, superficial. You just don't even want to talk to them. On the other hand, if they say, "Look, I don't really understand, but I have this amount of time, and I'd like to do something for you. Is there anything I can do for you practically?" Genuine interest, genuine concern—that's what helps. Just like everybody else wants, you know, genuine concern.

DR. KOENIG: What should friends and church members *not* do? You just said a little about that, go on . . .

JACKIE: Not try to fix you. Not try to condemn you. Not try to tell you that you don't have enough faith. Not be judgmental. Not think less of you . . . not treat you like an invalid. I hate being treated like an invalid.

DR. KOENIG: How can they not do that?

JACKIE: Just talk to you like—like you're normal, you know. Not like you're hard of hearing. You know, not like you're a child, or, "You poor thing."

DR. KOENIG: You don't want people to have pity?

JACKIE: No. That doesn't help anybody. Just be sincere.

DR. KOENIG: What could your husband do to help you with your pain?

JACKIE: He pretty much does it all, as I said before. He helps around the house. He helps with the housework, helps with the cooking, helps with the yard work.

DR. KOENIG: And what should he not do?

JACKIE: Pity. Grumble.

DR. KOENIG: What has helped you the most in coping with your pain?

JACKIE: Being able to go to God with it.

DR. KOENIG: Say a little bit more about that.

JACKIE: Being able to pray for other people, because it's not about me, it's about God. It's about what God wants me to do. Being able to allow Him to use my life in whatever's going on.

DR. KOENIG: Can you see any value for your pain, any good in your pain?

JACKIE: Yes. It causes me to recognize what's important in life. That it's not about things, and it's not about how much you have. It's about what you have and how you can allow God to use it, even in times when you feel insecure or unable. It's about allowing him to make you able.

DR. KOENIG: What about purpose in your pain?

JACKIE: The greatest purpose I guess is that in spite of what is going on, that I can still glorify Him and thank him for the life that He's given me. I guess it causes me to search God, to search the Word and find out what kind of relationship I can have with Him. It causes the relationship to be a lot more human than I could ever have had without the pain. I have a greater need to go to Him because of that pain.

DR. KOENIG: Has the pain brought you closer to God?

JACKIE: Yes. And I think it's caused my mind to grow and recognize more about what's going on outside of me, in the world.

DR. KOENIG: How has it done that?

JACKIE: It's made me more in touch with the purpose of things, and the purpose of life, and with people and their problems. It has helped me as a counselor to see how they can be healed, how to understand them and their situations better than I ordinarily would.

DR. KOENIG: The last question: What kind of advice would you have for other people like yourself with chronic pain?

JACKIE: Continue to trust God for healing the pain. It's not based on feelings. It's based on what the truth is. He promises us life and life abundantly. But he doesn't promise us a life without pain.

DR. KOENIG: Can you have abundant life if you have pain?

JACKIE: Yes, you can. I sure do.

Chapter 7

Long-Term Chronic Pain—Joan's Story

Joan, now age seventy-nine, has experienced chronic pain in her back and spine for over fifty years. She is a gracious, loving, and courageous person whom I have very much enjoyed having as a patient for the past five years. She has adapted to and accepted the pain, deciding to live a meaningful life in spite of the ongoing discomfort. She is a fiercely independent person, though, and has had difficulty asking for help (as have several others in previous chapters). This is the story of her life and how she has managed, especially now in her later years.

DR. KOENIG: When and where were you born?

JOAN: In Durham, North Carolina, July 29, 1921. I've lived there most of my life, except between the ages of two and twelve.

DR. KOENIG: Tell me about what it was like for you growing up.

JOAN: Growing up, really, I remember the Depression years. Being very proud of a new dress that was made out of three yards of material that cost ten cents a yard. What was it like in those days? Well, my parents had work, but no one really had a lot of work. They would work maybe one or two days a week. But we lived in a small town, and at the end of the street there was a lot of land and so my father had a huge garden where he raised our vegetables. And he raised hogs, so we had plenty of food.

DR. KOENIG: Was that after you left Durham?

JOAN: Yes, we left Durham when I was age two and lived in Roanoke Rapids until we moved back to Durham the summer I was twelve.

DR. KOENIG: What was your family life like when you were growing up?

JOAN: Both my parents had been married before, but each had lost their spouse to death. My father brought four children into the marriage. My mother had one child who died at an early age. My mother was an only child, and her mother lived with us and helped raise us. I didn't really get to know my mother until my grandmother contracted tuberculosis and was put into a sanitarium when I was about ten or eleven years old. My mother was a member of the Methodist church, and she sent us to Sunday school. But then, after my grandmother went into the sanitarium, we would spend Sundays visiting her there in Halifax, North Carolina, which was pretty far away. We would pack a lunch and maybe stop on the road and have lunch, and then go visit my grandmother in the afternoon, and then drive home. That was our routine until my grandmother died.

DR. KOENIG: And then you came back to Durham?

JOAN: Yes. We moved back to Durham the summer I was twelve. My oldest half sister was living here in Durham, and she attended the Baptist church, so I started to go with her to her church. But I just didn't fit in there. After a year or so, we moved to West Durham. Some friends of my father rented the parsonage for the Pentecostal Holiness Church. The house was attached to the church building. So we went with them to that church, and I had a wonderful Sunday school teacher, but again I just didn't fit in. I was in the eighth grade at school, I remember, and one of my classmates invited me to go with her to her Presbyterian church, and that's where I finally felt comfortable.

DR. KOENIG: How many years of schooling did you complete?

JOAN: I graduated from high school in 1939. My parents were of course too poor to send me on to college. Later I took a TV Bible course taught at University of North Carolina at Chapel Hill. I forget the professor's name, and as a matter of fact, we didn't even own a TV at the time. My next-door neighbor had a TV, and so we split the registration price. Then I missed one or two sessions because she had guests. So we bought our first TV so I could finish my Bible course. Later, I went to Durham Tech several times and took computer classes.

DR. KOENIG: What kind of a job or life aspirations did you have after getting out of school?

JOAN: Well, of course we were just coming out of the Depression years. My best friend got a job as the secretary to a doctor downtown at five dollars per week. My father was a supervisor in what was then called Erwin Mills [the same cotton mill where Bob's mom worked]. They had a strike at the mill, so my father told his superior that if he would promise me a job after the strike was over, he would let me work. So that was my first job and I stayed there until I married in 1943. I worked in the weaving section of the mill where they made sheeting material. On the end of the loom was what they called the battery where you placed the spools of cotton. Later I got a better job working with the weavers. When the weaver saw that there was an imperfection in the material, he would stop his loom, put a flag on it, and we would go and take a fine-toothed metal comb and pick out the bad spot so that he could start the loom again.

DR. KOENIG: How did you meet your husband?

JOAN: One late Sunday afternoon, I was on my front porch waiting for the time to go to church for our "Young People's" meeting. This car drove up in front of my house. Miss Betsy, our youth group leader, said, "Come on, and let's ride downtown." Of course I didn't know who she was with, but I learned his name was Fred. That's how I met my husband. It wasn't long, though, before he was called into the service (the last of January 1943), as World War II was starting. After writing to each other every day for almost six months, we were married in July of that year. We spent the night here in Durham and then left for Tennessee the next morning. That was on July 23, and I think it was in January 1944 that they moved him to Augusta, Georgia. We were not there too long before they moved him to California. And of course then it was during the war and we just didn't know what to expect, so I came home to stay with my parents in Durham.

DR. KOENIG: They transferred him to California?

JOAN: That's right. And then it looked like he was going to be there for awhile, so I took myself to California. After one month, they gave him leave to bring me home because he was being shipped overseas. He was sent to Germany for two years, and we corresponded daily during that time. He was in the Battle of the Bulge and there were six weeks during that battle that I didn't hear from him.

DR. KOENIG: And he made it through?

JOAN: Oh yes, with a little scar on the tip of his nose that, teasingly, I told him I thought was a girl's tooth print. It seems he was driving a truck laying communication wires, and something went wrong with the truck. So he went over to a downed airplane and pulled off a piece of aluminum to fix the truck, and it bounced back and hit him on the nose.

DR. KOENIG: What did you do during the two years he was overseas?

JOAN: I went back to the mill and worked there doing the same thing I had done before. When he came back from Germany after the war, we found a room in downtown Durham. Well, it was two rooms, I guess, behind the American Tobacco Company factory. It was so filthy. Also, we soon realized that when the factory let out at midnight there was a lot of noise, cars starting and blowing horns. We stayed there two weeks before finding a little three-room apartment on Guess Road. We stayed there until our first child was born, and then we moved to Cole Mill Road the day she was two months old in 1947.

DR. KOENIG: What kind of work did you do during your early marriage?

JOAN: I stayed at home with the first child. I didn't go back to work until after our second child was born four years later. Fred's cousin owned a cafeteria downtown. The girl that worked in his office either was getting married or was having a baby. Anyway, she was going to be away for a while and he asked me to fill in for her at the office while she was away. So I worked there at the cafeteria downtown until she came back.

DR. KOENIG: What did you do after that?

JOAN: Other opportunities soon opened. My sister-in-law was working at Duke University as a cashier in the cafeteria around that time. Because she lived on the other side of Durham and had a small child to take care of, it just became too much for her. So they asked her if she knew anyone that could take her place. School was just opening up, and it was a very bad time. She asked me if I could help out. I went to work as the cashier in the cafeteria, and worked in the office in between the meals. I ended up there for the next thirty-three years in the director's business office. My boss, it turns out, was head of food services for the U.S. Navy during World War II—the entire navy. And I mean, he knew his work. But he had that sailor's talk, and when he got mad, you surely knew about it.

DR. KOENIG: You worked there until you retired, is that correct?

JOAN: Yes, and I retired early because I was in bad health.

DR. KOENIG: Tell me about that. When did you first get injured?

JOAN: While Fred was in the service, my parents moved out to Broad Street near Guess Road. From the sidewalk out to my car, there were about two or three cement steps. I must have been in my mid-twenties when I tripped on one of those steps and fell and hurt my back. When the back pain didn't go away, I saw an orthopedic doctor. He just said that they didn't like to do surgery on women my age.

DR. KOENIG: What was the pain like?

JOAN: It just made me miserable. They treated it with a steel brace, and I wore that for two or three years before it just got to the point where I couldn't stand it anymore. And so they did the spinal fusion. I was around thirty years old at the time.

DR. KOENIG: Had you been working during this time?

JOAN: Yes, I had to work. Of course, I was in an office and sat in a chair, but I lived with a lot of pain.

DR. KOENIG: And how old are you now?

JOAN: I just had my seventy-ninth birthday last week.

DR. KOENIG: Let's move forward through time after the spinal fusion. Did your pain eventually get worse and cause you to retire finally after thirty years?

JOAN: There were a lot of changes occurring at Duke. The University food services had been under one person, but he left. Things then went from bad to worse. They just didn't find the right people to come in and run that big operation. It was getting on my nerves. I had moved to our office on East Campus and had to report to accounting in the Allen Building once a month. I would prepare the report and get it ready for the manager's signature. The report, however, was showing him in a bad light. And he would say, "Did you get this, did you get that?" And I would have to do the whole month's report over again and try to make him look better. It just got to be too much for me.

DR. KOENIG: So you resigned.

JOAN: I must have been about sixty-two, I think, and took early retirement.

DR. KOENIG: Was the psychological stress at work worse than the pain you were having?

JOAN: It was the two together. The pain, of course, was always there— and it's been there ever since I fell that first time.

DR. KOENIG: What is the pain like today?

JOAN: I still have back pain. I try to relieve it by sitting down in my La-Z-Boy chair that has a back massager. And maybe even put a heating pad on it. I do things like that before I break down and take pain medication.

DR. KOENIG: What limitations does the pain put on your life?

JOAN: I'm very limited these days. Since surgery a month ago, I haven't done much walking. That surgery wasn't on my back this time. I had a gallstone, the surgeon told my daughters, as large as a quarter.

DR. KOENIG: How does this pain, in your back and in your side, affect you on a day-to-day basis?

JOAN: Right now I'm just staying here in my little apartment most of the time. I don't get out much. I had to go pick up a refill for my medications this morning and just drove over to the pharmacy and back. I tried the heating pad for awhile but I had to take a pain pill.

DR. KOENIG: Where is most of the pain now?

JOAN: In the back.

DR. KOENIG: Do you have any trouble getting dressed in the morning or taking a shower?

JOAN: I haven't taken a shower in a long time. At home my shower was in the tub, and I was afraid I would fall. Since I've moved here, they have showers but my back won't allow me to stoop and sit down on the seat in the shower. So I'm just bathing from the sink.

DR. KOENIG: After you get dressed, how do you spend your day?

JOAN: I do a lot of sitting and reading. I brought my computer over here, but I haven't worked with it much. I'm sitting on my new bed right now. I paid twenty-five-hundred dollars for this bed just before I moved, but I'm still not able to sleep in it. I'm still sleeping in my La-Z-Boy chair.

DR. KOENIG: Do you also spend most of the afternoon sitting?

JOAN: Yes.

DR. KOENIG: What happens if you get up and walk around?

JOAN: Anytime I get moving, I get backaches. Right about where the surgery was done—in the lower back below the waist.

DR. KOENIG: And what is the pain like?

JOAN: Pressure I guess would be the best way to describe it. Deep, constant pressure. And the longer I stand on my feet, the stronger the pain gets.

DR. KOENIG: Does that pain ever interfere with your sleep at night?

JOAN: Yes, it does. Especially when I tried lying in this bed.

DR. KOENIG: How much sleep can you get before the pain wakes you up?

JOAN: I would say three to four hours. And then I get up. I don't know if you are familiar with it, but I watch a worship program that's on PAX TV, sometimes for hours. If I feel I can get back to sleep, then I just cut off the TV and go back to sleep. And occasionally I miss breakfast in the dining hall, but that's okay.

DR. KOENIG: Have pain medications helped your pain?

JOAN: Yes, they help. They don't do away with the pain, but it eases off enough so that you feel like you can live with it.

DR. KOENIG: What kind of medication do you take?

JOAN: Well, since this surgery, he's given me Percocet. Before that, I was taking Tylenol number three [with codeine] for my back.

DR. KOENIG: Concerning the surgery you had on your back years ago, did that help the pain?

JOAN: Oh yes, I couldn't have lived without the spinal fusion, I think. It was just too much pain. Before the surgery, it was just intolerable.

DR. KOENIG: Have you used any alternative medical treatments, natural substances, or other nonprescription pills or creams to help relieve your pain?

JOAN: I'm not much for buying medications without prescriptions because I just think there's a lot of fraud out there.

DR. KOENIG: The different herbs and vitamins that people take for pain—you don't take any of these?

JOAN: No, I don't. My husband's sister is a graduate of Duke's School of Nursing many years ago, and her husband graduated from Duke as well. When they left, he opened his neurology practice in Fort Lauderdale. So I have thought too much of people in the medical field to get into that [alternative medicine].

DR. KOENIG: How has the pain, day in and day out, affected you personally, and your feelings about yourself?

JOAN: I get nervous, you know. If I can't get the pain to ease off, then I just get really nervous. I don't know why.

DR. KOENIG: Do you look on yourself any differently because of your pain?

JOAN: No. I just realize that I have a problem that maybe some people don't have to deal with. But I think that is the only thing.

DR. KOENIG: How has the pain affected your family life, your time with your children?

JOAN: Well, of course it affects them. They realize that I am so limited in what I can do. Before, I was very active and just loved keeping house.

DR. KOENIG: Despite your back pain.

JOAN: Oh, absolutely.

DR. KOENIG: And when did you start becoming less active, such that it became a strain on your relationship with the children?

JOAN: I guess it was after I quit work about fifteen to twenty years ago that I really just gave into the pain for a long time. My family realized that I was in pain, and that I tried to do what I could to relieve it.

DR. KOENIG: What kinds of things did they want you to do that you couldn't do, that you had to say no to because of your limitations?

JOAN: Well, I guess I've always been just a homebody, even to begin with. Of course, I was very active in the church as long as I could, at Mount Bethel. In fact, Mount Bethel is a mission church from Blacknall Presbyterian, and I came out to Mount Bethel to help organize the young people many, many years ago.

DR. KOENIG: When did you have to stop your activity in the church?

JOAN: Four or five years ago. Before that, you know, I taught Sunday school. I was in the choir and did the office work at home (bulletins and newsletters) before we had an office at church.

DR. KOENIG: So church activity was one of the last activities you stopped doing?

JOAN: Absolutely. I even tried to start going again before Fred died, but I just couldn't. I'd go and take a cushion for my back. We were in a new sanctuary, and the pews—I just couldn't get comfortable. I've gone back in the past year or so to try again. But I was just so uncomfortable . . . I even sat near the back so that I could get up and leave and not disturb anyone, but I hated to do that. And I was just squirming, if you know what I mean. It was just too much. I didn't get anything out of the service because I was just so uncomfortable.

DR. KOENIG: And you took pain medication before you went?

JOAN: Yes, but it didn't help.

DR. KOENIG: How did your pain affect your relationship with your husband?

JOAN: I don't think that it made that much of a difference. I wore a TENS unit for awhile and that helped a great deal. As a matter of fact, I wore that when I was going to Durham Tech many years ago. But I couldn't put it on my back by myself. Fred did that for me as long as he could. I have a new TENS unit now, but I'm having trouble getting assistance to put it on.

DR. KOENIG: Did you take care of your husband Fred when he first got sick?

JOAN: Yes, Fred developed cancer, and then he had a heart attack. But it was the cancer that took him. And yes, I sat right up there in his room at Duke Hospital, slept in a chair for many nights there. He lost his voice and couldn't communicate, although he tried to "mouth" it.

DR. KOENIG: How long was he sick toward the end?

JOAN: Oh, perhaps, I'm afraid to say . . . maybe six months or longer. But there at the last, he'd open his mouth and say, "I want to go home. I want to go home." He couldn't utter a sound, but that's what he was trying to tell me. And so, there was nothing else they could do for him in the hospital. So I took him home about 6:00 p.m. one night, and he was there that night, and the next day, and then he died in the wee hours of the following morning. He's been gone five years this July fourth.

DR. KOENIG: How has the pain in your back affected you spiritually?

JOAN: It's brought me to my knees.

DR. KOENIG: Tell me about that.

JOAN: Well, I just talk to the Lord a lot. I guess that's my release.

DR. KOENIG: What kinds of questions do you ask God?

JOAN: I don't think it's so much asking questions, as asking Him to help me live with the pain. I think that's the main thing.

DR. KOENIG: You don't ever ask Him why you have it?

JOAN: No, no I don't. I have it, and I thank Him for the blessings that I do have. And ask Him to help me to live with the pain that I have.

DR. KOENIG: Did you ever ask God, why on earth, even as a young person, you had this pain?

JOAN: No.

DR. KOENIG: You just accepted it?

JOAN: Yes, yes. Well I knew that when I fell and hurt myself, they said they didn't want to do surgery on a person that young. And so I just learned to do the best I could with what I had.

DR. KOENIG: What could your friends or church members do to help with your pain?

JOAN: They often ask me, "What can I do to help you?" Well, of course, when I was living at home I got to the place where I couldn't keep the house. They were willing to come in, but I didn't ask them to. Everybody has their own problems and pain, and I just felt like I didn't want to ask them to come in.

DR. KOENIG: But you could have used their help?

JOAN: Yes, I could have. But I would have felt uncomfortable for them to come in and do the things that needed to be done. I had a housekeeper who came in to do the house, until she got so old she couldn't. And nowadays, you know, in Durham, when you're a woman living alone, you just can't let strangers come in. And so the house was not being kept the way I like my home to be kept toward the end of the time I lived there.

DR. KOENIG: But even though people offered, you still didn't feel right letting them come in and help?

JOAN: Actually they came. . . . After hurricane Fran, a group of men came from the church and cleaned up the yard as much as they could.

DR. KOENIG: So church members could offer to do things, and perhaps in a really difficult situation they could actually help out?

JOAN: Yes, and maybe there are some people who would not have trouble accepting it. I just wanted to be the giver, not the receiver.

DR. KOENIG: What else could church members do, say emotionally, that would lift you up and make you feel better?

JOAN: Well, up until the last year, we had prayer chains, and I headed up one of the prayer chains. There were many things going on in the church where people needed prayer. I'm still doing that—I still get calls for prayer help. But it's automatic, now, on the phone—the telephone automatically dials everyone on the chain and tells them about the prayer needs.

DR. KOENIG: When did you stop directing the prayer chain?

JOAN: When they put it on automatic from the office, about nine months ago. It tells who it is that needs prayer and why. Before it went automatic, we actually got so many calls that we broke it down into three chains, one of which I headed up. I would call one person, and they would call the next, and so forth. The last one would call me back to be sure that the chain had not been broken.

DR. KOENIG: Being part of that prayer chain was helpful.

JOAN: Oh yes, and then too, Mount Bethel had grown and is still growing. There are so many people there I didn't know, and even though it was only on the phone, I got to meet some of the newer members that way.

DR. KOENIG: How else might church members help?

JOAN: Well, I think at least offering to help, even though, like me, I decided not to accept the offer. Offer to help. A card now and then or a phone call would certainly let you know that they are thinking about you.

DR. KOENIG: What about your family? What could your family do to help you with your pain? Do you have children that live nearby?

JOAN: I have two girls. Jill will be fifty-three in September, and Sandy is forty-nine. Only one of them lives here in Durham, but her husband left her in a very bad way, and that poor girl is working three jobs to make a living. So she does what she can.

DR. KOENIG: If it weren't for those limitations, how could your daughters help?

JOAN: Well, they could think of things that I wouldn't think about that might need to be done. Honestly, I was so surprised the other day. My birthday was last Saturday. When I opened the door in the morning to go down for breakfast and there was this beautiful balloon saying, "Happy Birthday," tied around the knocker on my door. That was the most pleasant surprise. And so when my daughter called, I said, "Did you come down here this morning?" It seems that she came by here about 10:00 p.m. the night before. "I'm just going up to tie this balloon on her door and I'll be right back down," she said to the attendant. I hear noises out in the hall sometimes. And I did that night. I heard her, but it never dawned on me what was going on. So I looked and saw that I hadn't locked my door. And she was standing right there when I locked the door!

DR. KOENIG: So doing little surprises for you like this really helps. Anything else?

JOAN: Yes, phone calls really help. Just hearing their voice and learning about what they're doing.

DR. KOENIG: When you think of all of the things that have helped you cope with pain, day in and day out, what has helped you the most?

JOAN: Well, I do think painkillers help. I have a healthy respect for them and I try to be very careful in using them. As I said before, first I'll use the vibrator on my back. Then I use the heating pad. I'll try everything else to ease the pain before I take medication.

DR. KOENIG: What helps you the most in coping emotionally with the kind of depression or frustration that this pain causes?

JOAN: Probably reading, get involved in something so I can sort of forget about the pain. Get my mind on something else.

DR. KOENIG: Can you see any value in your pain?

JOAN: No. Unless maybe it makes me humble. I realize that I'm not able to do what I would really like to do. I'd like to be more active but I can't be.

DR. KOENIG: When you say humble, humble with respect to . . .

JOAN: Realizing that there is a power greater than I, and that I'm limited.

DR. KOENIG: Has your pain brought you closer to God?

JOAN: Oh, I'm sure. I can't imagine anyone living with what I'm living with if they didn't have the Lord.

DR. KOENIG: So you feel like you've grown closer to God because of your pain?

JOAN: I'm sure He knows me!

DR. KOENIG: If you never had one bit of pain in your life, do you think you would be as close to Him?

JOAN: Probably not. As I said, my mother started me as a child in Sunday school, so I've been going to church all my life. I can't even imagine what it would be like without Him.

DR. KOENIG: Going to church and participating in different religious activities are one thing, but getting to know God, that's different isn't it?

JOAN: Yes, it is. I've come to know Him personally, and as I said, I'm sure He knows me too.

DR. KOENIG: What advice would you have for other people like yourself, in chronic pain?

JOAN: Well, I would first say to seek medical help. There may be something that can relieve it. So try to get relief medically. And then, if you cannot get relief, you just have to work around it.

DR. KOENIG: What about coping emotionally with the pain?

JOAN: Praying, probably.

DR. KOENIG: That's what you've done?

JOAN: That's what I've done and what I'm still doing.

Chapter 8

Assessment of Pain

CONSEQUENCES OF PAIN

The preceding stories about people in pain should give the reader a glimpse of how severe, unrelenting pain can affect an individual physically, emotionally, socially, behaviorally, and spiritually. Experiencing pain day in and day out, month after month, sometimes year after year, slowly wears down the person in each of these domains.

Constant physical discomfort is physically exhausting. Imagine the continual experience of sensations of burning, shooting, tearing, squeezing, or boring discomfort that sometimes escalates to the point of complete immobilization of the person with nauseating agony (as occurred with Bob and Penny). Pain of high intensity is accompanied by an urge to escape the intolerable feeling. Pain forces a person's attention to it, making it difficult to concentrate on anything else. This focused attention then heightens the pain sensations, which further increase the desire to escape from it.

Efforts to relieve the pain are often directed at decreasing activity. Some with severe pain even develop a fear of movement called kinesophobia.[1] Attempts to reduce or stop movement result in deconditioning, with loss of muscle mass and strength, increased rigidity of ligaments, and reduced bone density. Reduced activity also increases the likelihood of weight gain, which may further exacerbate pain and decrease the ability to move about. For some persons, eating is the only pleasure they have left. Uncontrolled appetite, however, results in further weight problems that increase pain with movement and reinforce immobility. Reduced ability to concentrate, decreased activity, and increased weight often carry the person downward in a vicious cycle of increasing disability and dependency.

Because pain forces the sufferer to pay attention to it, it often interferes with sleep and rest at night. The person with chronic pain may shift and turn repeatedly to get into a more comfortable position that will at least temporarily ease the discomfort. Difficulty sleeping is associated with daytime fatigue and exhaustion that drain a person's emotional resources, making him or her more irritable, frustrated, and prone to outbursts of anger over minor difficulties.

Fear and anxiety are other common emotions that accompany chronic pain (as Laura and Joan experienced). When people are in pain, they often worry about whether relief will ever come. If relief does come, then they worry about when the pain will return. The near-constant attention paid to the pain or attempts to relieve it drain the joy and happiness out of life, and quickly bring on feelings of helplessness and despair.

Feelings of loneliness also quickly follow, along with the sense that others don't really understand what it is like to have chronic pain unless they too are experiencing it. Furthermore, since pain complaints often cannot be objectively verified and create increased burdens on others, the result is that friends, loved ones, or caregivers may doubt whether the person is really having as much pain as he or she claims. Perhaps the person is exaggerating the pain, or the pain is all in his or her head. This lack of understanding and failure of others to believe them further forces sufferers to retreat into their own isolated world. They often feel abandoned by their physician, caretaker, family, friends, and sometimes even by God.

It is easy, then, for the person to feel that there is no way out of these circumstances; to stop trying and give up. Feeling trapped, locked into an intolerable existence characterized by physical, emotional, and spiritual pain, a person loses hope and depression quickly ensues. Little wonder then why so many either numb themselves with drugs or alcohol, or when that fails, attempt suicide. Pain is serious business.

ASSESSMENT

For these reasons, the assessment of pain has become a mandate in doctor's offices and hospitals around the country. It is no longer optional. Recall that JCAHO is now requiring that people have their pain assessed and managed appropriately; if a health care institution fails to do so, its licensure may be revoked. Pain is quickly becoming the "fifth vital sign" in terms of routine assessment (along with pulse, blood pressure, temperature, and respiratory rate).[2] Common sense dictates that determining the cause of the pain is necessary for the doctor to choose the right treatment. Two people may have identical pain complaints, but have completely different causes requiring different treatments (for example, someone with a tension headache versus someone with a migraine). Thus, before a doctor can develop a plan of treatment, he or she must take a comprehensive history of the pain.[3] It is important to know what kind of information is useful to the doctor when providing a pain history.

Description

The pain should be described to the doctor in the patient's own words. What is the pain like? Is it a burning pain, a shooting pain, or a pain that feels like a jolt of electricity (e.g., neuropathic pain)? Is it a stabbing, penetrating, boring kind of pain? Is it a sore, aching, deep, constant pain (e.g., arthritic pain)? Is the pain best characterized as a heaviness or tightness (as in cardiac pain or esophageal spasm)? Does the pain come on gradually, build to a crescendo, and then slowly ease off (e.g., intestinal or ureteral spasm)? Does the pain come on suddenly and leave suddenly, or is it constant and present all the time?

Severity

The gold standard for assessing pain severity is the report provided by the patient. Severity is best assessed using a verbal rating scale (mild, moderate, severe), or may be determined by asking the person to rate on a zero to ten numerical scale how bad the pain is—where zero means "no pain at all" and ten means "the most severe pain ever experienced." This is the most common way that doctors and other health professionals assess pain.[4] It is simple and reliable. When I had my kidney stone attack, the doctors monitored my pain level using this zero to ten scale, and despite the effects of the pain on my concentration, I was able to accurately and quickly convey to the physicians how bad the pain was. It is important to measure and document the severity of pain from one time to another, both to assess whether pain treatments are working and to determine if the disease causing the pain is getting worse.

Besides the simple zero-to-ten pain scale, the shortest and most widely used instrument for measuring pain, the McGill Pain Questionnaire, consists of fifteen adjectives that describe the quality of the pain and associated emotional suffering.[5] There is a longer version of the McGill Pain Questionnaire often used in research studies that assesses pain severity, location, and characteristics using twenty different descriptors.[6]

Unfortunately, there are no objective, biological markers or blood tests to document the presence or the severity of pain. The most accurate and reliable method of determining the intensity of pain is to simply ask the person how bad the pain is.[7] Consequently, experts recommend that people's complaints of pain be taken seriously. This is particularly true for chronic pain that is often exhausting and associated with a multiplicity of physical, mental, and social consequences.[8]

Location and Duration

Where is the pain located? Can the pain be pinpointed to a specific location, or is it more diffuse and difficult to localize? Does it radiate or extend out from one body part to another (i.e., from the low back down into the leg or foot)? Does it feel more superficial, or near or on the skin (such as a burn), or deeper in the muscles or bone (such as blunt trauma)? Does it occur only on one side of the body, or is it symmetrical and present equally on both sides? The answers to these questions give the doctor clues that will help him or her identify the cause of the pain.

How long has the pain persisted—a few hours, days, months, or years? What were the circumstances in which it arose? Did it start after an accident, fall, or specific incident, or did it arise on its own without any precipitating cause? If a precipitating event can be identified, the cause of the pain is much more easy to determine.

What is the relationship with activity? Does activity worsen or improve the pain? What kinds of activity worsen the pain? Do certain activities relieve the pain? Does standing, sitting, or lying down in a particular position relieve or worsen the pain? What activities has the person given up because of the pain? Are there any plans for increased activity should the pain lessen?

Effects on Personal Relationships

How has the pain affected relationships with friends or those at work? What about family members and loved ones? Does it interfere when playing with children? How does it affect the relationship with a husband or wife? Does the pain interfere with religious activities such as going to church or participating in church-related social events? Have there been other problems associated with the pain such as psychological symptoms, decline in ability to carry out responsibilities, spiritual distress, existential distress, financial worries, or related concerns? These questions are crucial for determining the overall impact of the pain on the person's life.

Previous History of Pain

Is there a history of pain prior to the current pain? If so, was that pain similar to the pain now? How was it similar? How was it different? How did the pain arise? Was a doctor consulted, and what was the diagnosis? What types of remedies were used to treat the pain and how effective were they?

Treatments for Pain

Have appropriate interventions been taken to relieve the pain? Has the person seen a doctor for the pain recently? Is he or she taking medication? What kinds of medication seem to help? Which medicines have not helped? Has the person had surgery for the pain or had any other procedure (nerve block, spinal fusion, etc.)? What about the use of complementary or alternative therapies for the pain, such as acupuncture, spinal manipulation, or other nontraditional treatments? Has the person tried vitamins or over-the-counter natural or herbal pain remedies, applied magnets for relief, or utilized other unusual or lesser-known methods to reduce the pain? Such information is important for the doctor to know as he or she develops a treatment plan for the pain.

Physical Examination

After taking a complete history, the doctor should conduct a careful physical examination not just of the painful part, but also of the entire physical body, since problems in the body far away from the pain may be the cause of the pain (for example, knee pain may result from damage to the hip joint). The physical should include a detailed neurological examination that tests sensation to pain, heat, cold, vibration, and light touch, muscle strength and coordination, reflexes, and gait (how the patient walks), searching for any asymmetries that may be present. The physical exam is then often followed by blood tests, X rays, CT or MRI scans, and perhaps by nerve conduction studies or electromyograms.

KEY CONSIDERATIONS DURING ASSESSMENT

When assessing pain, the doctor must consider a number of important factors. First, what degree of underlying disease or physical damage is present? Are there diseases that could explain the pain? Every effort must be made to identify an underlying organic or biological basis for the pain. Pain is usually a signal that there is ongoing tissue damage which requires attention. A comprehensive medical and neurological evaluation as described previously is necessary to rule out any possible physical causes for the pain, especially those for which there is available treatment.

Second, is there evidence in the person's history or in his or her interaction with the doctor that symptoms are being amplified for psychological or social gain, whether intentionally or unintentionally? Does the patient display pain behaviors such as grimacing, rigidity, or guarded movements? Because pain is a subjective phenomenon (dependent on the person's own report), people may either consciously or unconsciously take advantage of this to elicit nurturance, attention, or financial gain. Is the person undergoing litigation related to the pain? Is he or she currently receiving disability compensation? If the pain were to improve, would he or she have a job waiting? Is there a history of frequent job changes or long periods without work prior to the onset of the pain? All of these factors influence both the perception and the report of pain. In some cases, the potential gains from having the pain are so high that the person may not be aware that these are affecting his or her motivation toward recovery. Such motivation is also affected by the presence of other family members with chronic pain, since they provide comfortable role models.

Third, are there psychosocial issues present that complicate the pain presentation? During the assessment, the health care professional must ask the patient about depression or suicidal thoughts. Were major stressors present in the patient's life before pain began or worsened, and have any occurred since that time? Is there a high level of marital or family conflict and dissatisfaction? If so, did this arise before or after the pain began?

Finally, what are the expectations of the health care provider? Are these expectations realistic or unrealistic? Is the expectation total relief of all pain? Is the expectation just to obtain help in coping with the pain? Are medication, surgery, behavioral, or psychosocial treatments expected? This information will impact satisfaction and compliance with the prescribed therapy.

OVERCOMING BARRIERS TO PAIN ASSESSMENT

According to a 1998 consensus panel convened by the American Geriatrics Society,[9] numerous barriers prevent adequate assessment of pain. Although this report focused on older adults, it applies to persons of all ages. Barriers include a reluctance to report pain, a denial of pain, and difficulty with communication. Older adults may expect pain with aging or describe their pain in terms of "aching" or "discomfort," which tend to minimize the complaint. Many persons may deny having pain for fear that they have a serious disease. With older adults, difficulty with communication may interfere with reports of pain, especially in those individuals with dementia or hearing problems.

There are several things that physicians can do to overcome barriers to pain assessment. When doctors ask about pain, they should always include in their inquiry such words as *burning, aching, soreness, heaviness,* or *tightness,* which are likely to help identify pain complaints that otherwise might not be mentioned. Any persistent pain that interferes with a person's ability to function at work or at home, or that otherwise impairs quality of life, should be taken seriously and treated. Nonverbal pain behavior (agitation, restlessness, withdrawal) should be looked for in people with communication problems. Collateral sources of information should be sought, including reports from family members or caregivers.

IS THE PAIN REAL?

The clinician's attitude toward the patient during the process of assessing chronic pain is extremely important for an effective and sensitive evaluation. Most experts agree that unless there are strong reasons to the contrary, the doctor should believe the patient's report concerning the reality and seriousness of the pain, since it is better to err in the direction of overdiagnosing pain than discounting the complaints of even a few true sufferers. Furthermore, as previously noted, pain is a highly complex biological, psychological, and social experience that scientists are just beginning to understand. Recent research is uncovering just how complex the phenomenon of chronic pain really is.

At a recent annual meeting of the American Association for the Advancement of Science in Washington, DC, scientists described advances in the understanding of pain.[10] Many presenters argued that chronic pain should be viewed as a disease, not just a symptom. According to Dr. Alan Basbaum from the University of California, San Francisco, "persistent pain is in fact a disease. Many of the changes that occur actually occur at the level of the spinal cord, and it occurs in some respects by the establishment of memories of pain, memories of the injury, long-lasting memories." He emphasized that in addition to pain occurring at the site of injury, pain was also in the brain. Other presenters noted that in studies of mice, 50 percent of the variability in pain threshold was determined by genetic factors. Using brain imaging, Dr. Catherine Bushnell of McGill University in Montreal, Canada, reported that persons who experience injury to the spinal cord or central nervous system that causes chronic pain have a "reorganization of the sensory part of the cortex that appears to be maintained by the pain."

Similarly, researchers at Washington University School of Medicine in St. Louis, Missouri, have discovered that normally "silent" cells in the spinal cord may lead to chronic pain.[11] Some cells located in the dorsal horn of the spinal cord that normally do not participate in pain messages may become activated under conditions of intense or persistent pain so that the cells then begin sending pain signals to the brain. Once activated, however, these nerves become so efficient at sending pain messages that they continue to do this even after healing has occurred. This may help to explain why some people experience chronic pain even after healing of the original injury is complete. Such persons may experience pain even when touched only very lightly (called allodynia). Why would the body have developed such a mechanism? Perhaps, study researchers hypothesized, "If an animal is injured, it does not want a second injury, so it may facilitate (pain signals) not only at the injury site, but at other sites."[12]

If a good percentage of our sensitivity to pain is determined by our genetic makeup or our sensitivity to objective changes caused by pain in the nervous system, these facts may go a long way toward destigmatizing pain. As doctors assess and evaluate people with chronic pain, such factors should be kept in mind. Even if no objective cause for pain can be identified, there may be biological factors responsible for it.

SUMMARY AND CONCLUSIONS

Chronic pain may come from many different sources. The cause of the pain will often determine the best and most effective treatment. For that reason, a comprehensive medical, neurological, and psychological assessment is essential. When assessing someone in pain, the doctor should ask about the intensity, character, frequency, location, duration, and precipitants of pain, and also about what relieves the pain. The doctor should also conduct a comprehensive physical examination looking for neurological deficits, weaknesses, increased sensation, numbness, or other unusual sensations or lack of sensation. The person should be assessed for functional abilities that the pain may be interfering with, such as standing, walking, reaching, and turning. Doctors should ask about psychosocial functioning, including assessment of family and social relationships. All patients with pain should be assessed for complications related to the pain—depression, drug or alcohol addiction—and treatment should be initiated for these problems. Finally, it is important to assess for any motivational factors that may be influencing the presentation of pain, and to determine what the person's expectations are concerning treatment.

People with chronic pain and their family members should expect such a comprehensive evaluation from their medical doctors. If most of these elements are not present in the pain evaluation, then missing elements should be brought to the attention of the physician. This will increase the likelihood that the doctor will diagnose the correct cause of the pain and prescribe the most appropriate and effective treatment.

Chapter 9

Medication for Pain

I didn't realize how important it was to relieve pain until I recently experienced the pain of a kidney stone. This occurred suddenly one morning after a speaking engagement in Clearwater, Florida. For what seemed like eternity I endured excruciating pain as I had never experienced before. After hours of praying with my wife over the situation, I realized that the pain was not going away. We then called 911, and I was transported to the nearest emergency room for treatment. During the next several hours, while the doctors were investigating the cause of my pain, they could not give me any pain relief for fear of disguising the symptoms. I was writhing in agony, unable to find a position that would ease the pain, pain that was being made worse by all the diagnostic tests and X rays. The cause for the pain was identified as a stone blocking my right ureter resulting in the obstruction and subsequent rupture of my right kidney. After nearly seven hours, I was finally given a shot of meperidine (Demerol) and promethazine (Phenergan), and the pain began to ease off. What joy and sense of relief I felt to lose that pain.

Although I had been a practicing physician for twenty years, it was not until then that I truly realized how important it was for doctors to take their patients' pain complaints seriously and do whatever is necessary to relieve that pain. As indicated in Chapter 8, unrelieved pain over time may actually rewire the nervous system until it becomes hypersensitive to pain, which becomes more difficult to treat. The adequate treatment of pain right from the start, then, becomes absolutely essential. On the other hand, excessive use of pain medication may result in serious side effects, irreversible organ damage, and the development of tolerance, physical dependence, and in some cases, addiction. It is important, then, to know something about the pain medications that are available and how to use them effectively.

The type of medicine used for the treatment of pain differs depending on whether the pain is acute (sudden, severe, but time limited—as was my kidney stone), chronic (continuous or recurrent and long-standing—such as arthritis), or due to a disease process such as cancer that ends in death.[1] (Chapter 13 will discuss the management of cancer-related pain.) Little is mentioned here about medications for acute pain due to an injury, time-limited disease process, or surgical operation, since these treatments are similar to medication used for chronic pain particularly during short periods of acute worsening. The most notable difference between the treatment of acute and chronic pain is that narcotic pain relievers are more readily given for acute pain since they need to be given only for a short while.

For acute pain, doctors prescribe medications ranging in potency from acetaminophen (Tylenol) or acetylsalicylic acid (aspirin) to opium-derived drugs such as morphine or meperidine (narcotic pain relievers). Narcotics may be administered by intramuscular or even intravenous injection. If pain is severe and not relieved by a single medicine, combinations of medication may be tried—for example, including an antinausea or antianxiety drug that may boost the effects of the pain reliever. Despite widespread fears that taking narcotic pain relievers can cause addiction, studies have shown that many people with severe, acute physical pain who take narcotic analgesics do not experience excessive sedation or a need to continuously increase their dose. Finding the optimal medication dose, not too much or too little for the amount of pain present, can be a fine art and may require skillful dosage adjustments.

MEDICATING CHRONIC PAIN

In the rest of this chapter, I discuss medication for chronic pain due to conditions such as arthritis, low back problems, fibromyalgia, neuropathic pain syndromes, phantom limb pain, central pain syndrome, protracted pain from injury or burns, neuralgias, headaches, and other nonmalignant causes of long-term pain (lasting three months or longer). As noted earlier, chronic pain may be associated with ongoing tissue damage, may continue after initial healing has taken place, or may occur in the absence of any objective evidence of tissue damage. Although medication guidelines for the treatment of acute pain, postoperative pain, and cancer pain have been developed by the Agency for Health Care Policy and Research (AHCPR) and by the American Pain Society, relatively little attention has been paid to the treatment of chronic noncancer pain that is so widespread today.[2]

A different treatment strategy must be taken for chronic pain than for acute pain. This is particularly true when chronic pain is initially treated with narcotic analgesics. This is because of the development of tolerance and physical dependence that occurs when narcotics are used over an extended time period. In other words, when people take narcotic pain relievers for weeks or months, their bodies tend to get used to the medication and they have to take more and more medication to get the same level of pain relief. Soon the body builds up such a resistance to the pain medication that even large doses of medication lose their effectiveness in relieving pain. Furthermore, narcotic pain relievers often have unpleasant side effects that may not improve even after weeks or months of taking the drug. These side effects include difficulty concentrating, worsening constipation, and excessive sedation. Therefore, a medication used for chronic pain should be one that has relatively few side effects and will be effective for relieving pain in the long term without needing to continuously increase the dose.

Chronic pain is complicated by emotional and psychological factors more often than acute pain. Chronic pain may begin with a physical cause, but psychological factors may start playing a role in the pain as it continues relentlessly over months and months. The treatment of chronic pain differs from acute pain in that chronic pain therapies should follow a rehabilitative model rather than an acute treatment model (although they are not mutually exclusive). The term *rehabilitation* means the chronic pain sufferer learns to accept and adapt his or her life to the pain, relying less on medication and more on activities that lessen the pain or reduce its psychological consequences.

Chronic pain clinics are based on this rehabilitative model. In these clinics, medical doctors who specialize in the treatment of pain help individuals to reduce their dosages of narcotic medication, and institute a regimen of exercise, relaxation, and diet to help counteract the associated inactivity and depression. Relaxation techniques include hypnosis, biofeedback, and meditation. Traditional Christian prayer can also be utilized. Certain devices may be used to interrupt the pain signal in or near the spinal cord. One such device is called a transcutaneous electronic nerve stimulator (more on this and other mechanical therapies in Chapter 12).

In chronic pain, every effort should be made to optimize treatment of the underlying disease causing the pain.[3] In other words, if someone is having chronic chest pain due to insufficient blood supply to the heart from coronary artery blockages, every effort should be made to relieve the obstructions by medication or surgery. Likewise, if someone is experiencing knee pain because of joint inflammation, an anti-inflammatory drug should be taken to reduce the swelling and pain, or if extensive joint destruction has already taken place, a total knee operation should be performed. Unfortunately, there are no treatments for the underlying causes of many types of chronic pain such as osteoarthritis or neuropathic pain, and treatment of unpleasant symptoms with pain relievers may be the only treatment possible. Pharmacological therapies for chronic pain are described in the paragraphs that follow, beginning with the most benign treatments with the fewest side effects and progressing to drugs that are more risky. See Tables 1 through 3 in Appendix II for more details about administration and side effects of specific medications.

NONNARCOTIC ANALGESICS

Acetaminophen

The treatment of first choice for chronic pain is acetaminophen (Tylenol). Almost all people with chronic pain should start out on a scheduled dose of acetaminophen, taking it regularly three or four times per day. The maximum safe dose of acetaminophen is 4,000 milligrams (mg) per day for adults. This is equivalent to taking two 500 mg tablets of acetaminophen (Extra-Strength Tylenol) every six hours, or four 325 mg tablets (regular Tylenol) every eight hours. Persons with pre-existing liver disease, a history of heavy alcohol use, or severe physical debility should take less than the 4,000 mg/day limit. At doses higher than 4,000 mg/day, the risk of liver damage increases. Acetaminophen has only analgesic (pain-relieving) effects and no anti-inflammatory properties; it will not improve inflammation if that is what is causing pain (as in rheumatoid and other inflammatory kinds of arthritis).

For some reason, people are often reluctant to take acetaminophen, particularly at high doses such as those described here. Nevertheless, pain experts uniformly agree that high-dose acetaminophen should be the first intervention for treating people with chronic pain. It is also the safest, has almost no side effects, and has no potential for physical dependence or addiction.

Aspirin

Aspirin is an extremely effective pain reliever and anti-inflammatory drug. Two 325 mg aspirin (total 650 mg) tablets every four to six hours provide relatively powerful pain relief and anti-inflammatory effects. The total dose taken each day may be increased until just below that level which causes a "ringing" sound in the ears. The side effects associated with aspirin use, especially high-dose aspirin (twelve tablets per day), are significant and include gastrointestinal irritation and bleeding, increased bruising and bleeding elsewhere, and possibly disorientation at higher doses. Aspirin is a type of nonsteroidal anti-inflammatory drug (NSAIDs) and in fact was the first drug in this class to appear on the market.

Combinations

A number of over-the-counter pain relievers can be purchased at local drugstores or grocery stores. Many of these involve combinations of acetaminophen or aspirin, together with caffeine. Excedrin, Anacin, and BC powder are common examples. These are no more effective than standard doses of either acetaminophen or aspirin, particularly when these drugs are taken on a regular schedule throughout the day; furthermore, the inclusion of other substances such as caffeine complicates their use.

NSAIDs

NSAIDs are a relatively safe class of drugs for chronic pain, although side effects are greater than for acetaminophen and possibly even aspirin. NSAIDs work by reducing prostaglandin synthesis. Prostaglandins are hormonelike substances that increase in body tissues whenever there is an injury (whether caused by external trauma or by destructive internal autoimmune processes such as arthritis). Prostaglandins play an important role in causing inflammation and pain. NSAIDs reduce prostaglandin synthesis by interfering with the activity of two enzymes, cyclo-oxygenase 1 and cyclo-oxygenase 2, necessary for its production. Each of these two enzymes has a specific job in the body. Cyclo-oxygenase 1 plays an important role in the normal functioning of the kidney and liver, whereas cyclo-oxygenase 2 is the culprit primarily responsible for inflammation and pain. It is important to distinguish the activity of these two enzymes. Until recently most of the NSAIDs impaired *both* enzymes, resulting in reduction of inflammation (from cyclo-oxygenase 2 inhibition) and worrisome kidney and gastrointestinal side effects (from cyclo-oxygenase 1 inhibition).

Serious side effects caused by NSAIDs result in 100,000 hospitalizations and 17,000 deaths each year.[4] About 1 percent of people in the general population experience gastrointestinal bleeding when they take NSAIDs such as Motrin or Aleve, a rate that increases to 3 to 4 percent in persons over age sixty, and up to 9 percent in those with a history of gastrointestinal bleeding from ulcers or stomach irritation.[5] This side effect can be partially but not totally relieved by taking medicines such as misoprostol (Cytotec), histamine receptor antagonists (Zantac or Pepcid), or antacids (Maalox or Mylanta). Likewise, impairment of kidney function is a real concern, particularly if NSAIDs are used over an extended time period. All NSAIDs currently on the market can cause these potential complications. Rather than expose patients to these side effects, some doctors would rather prescribe low-dose opioid (narcotic) analgesics, low-dose corticosteroid therapy (if inflammation is the problem), or combination drug therapies (pain relievers plus antidepressants or anticonvulsants) rather than risk long-term NSAID use.

In order to function, I've had to take NSAIDs regularly since I was about thirty years old. I've taken several of these drugs, including tolmetin (Tolectin), high-dose aspirin, and flurbiprofen (Ansaid). I'd take one drug for several years and then for some reason it would slowly lose its effectiveness. Interestingly, naproxen (Naprosyn) and ibuprofen (Motrin) never worked very well for me. That's a funny thing about NSAIDs—different people have different responses to any one particular drug in this class. Luckily, I have thus far not had gastrointestinal or kidney problems on these drugs, although it is a constant worry. Doctors have ways of monitoring people who take NSAIDs to detect these side effects early. Tests commonly conducted for this purpose include checking feces for blood due to gastrointestinal bleeding or irritation (the stool guaiac test) and drawing blood for tests of kidney (serum creatinine) and liver function. My doctor performs these tests once a year on me. I'm thankful that drug companies are working fervently to develop new anti-inflammatory drugs that are more effective and have fewer side effects.

COX-2 Inhibitors

The latest breakthroughs in the search for new drugs to treat chronic pain include selective cyclo-oxygenase 2 (COX-2) inhibitors such as celecoxib (Celebrex), rofecoxib (Vioxx), and meloxicam (M-cam or Mobic). These drugs block only cyclo-oxygenase 2, the enzyme responsible for pain-related inflammation, while sparing to some degree cyclo-oxygenase 1, the enzyme necessary for stomach, kidney, and liver function. None of the drugs indicated, however, block only the COX-2 enzyme, so some people still have stomach and kidney problems while taking these drugs.[6] The "next generation" of cyclo-oxygenase-inhibiting drugs now being developed by drug companies will be more selective for the COX-2 enzyme, further reducing unwanted side effects by preserving the function of the COX-1 enzyme.

Two years ago I began taking COX-2 inhibitors. First I tried Celebrex. It was very effective, but because of an allergy to sulfa drugs, I developed an allergic reaction to that medication (severe inflammation of the muscles in my upper arms and thighs) and had to stop. I then began taking Vioxx, which has been very effective thus far in controlling the pain and inflammation caused by psoriatic arthritis. I've been trying to slowly reduce my dose so that I take only the minimal amount necessary to control my symptoms and allow me to function. When I first started Vioxx, I took 25 mg once in the morning and 25 mg once in the evening. About six months ago I reduced it to 25 mg in the morning and 12.5 mg in the evening, and recently I've reduced it to just 25 mg at night (which is still effective). There is some evidence that Vioxx may be more effective than Celebrex for pain from osteoarthritis.[7]

Antidepressants

For some time now, doctors have known that treating chronic pain with low doses of antidepressant medication seems to ease the pain.[8] A review of thirty-nine carefully controlled clinical trials on the analgesic effects of antidepressants in chronic pain found that patients receiving an antidepressant reported less pain than 74 percent of patients receiving a placebo.[9] Another review of eleven studies found that treatment with antidepressants resulted in a significant reduction in pain compared with placebo even in patients with psychogenic pain or somatoform pain disorder.[10] Research suggests that antidepressants not only affect pain by treating depression, providing sedation, and causing a placebo effect but also by a direct analgesic action.[11]

Most of the scientific evidence that supports the effectiveness of antidepressants for pain relief involves the use of tricyclic antidepressants. Antidepressants in this drug class unfortunately have a host of unpleasant side effects that may include constipation, difficulty urinating, dizziness, visual changes, dry mouth, blood pressure changes, heart rhythm irregularities, and other physical or mental effects. Newer antidepressants such as fluoxetine (Prozac), called selective serotonin reuptake inhibitors (SSRIs), while having fewer side effects, may not be as effective as tricyclic antidepressants in relieving pain.[12]

Low-dose tricyclic antidepressants such as amitriptyline (Elavil) (10 to 25 mg/day) or nortriptyline (Pamelor) (10 to 20 mg/day) can be used either alone or in combination with other analgesics to help relieve pain. Besides providing sedation and facilitating sleep at night, these drugs are believed to act directly on the central nervous system pain centers, reducing their responsivity to pain impulses. Tricyclic antidepressants may be especially helpful for fibromyalgia or diabetic neuropathy. The combination of an SSRI (fluoxetine, 20 mg) and a tricyclic (amitriptyline, 25 mg) may be particularly beneficial in persons struggling with fibromyalgia.[13]

One of my colleagues at Duke University, Dr. Veerainder Goli, recently discovered that the antidepressant venlafaxine (Effexor XR) may be an effective treatment for chronic pain due to diabetic neuropathy.[14] Many people with diabetes experience severe pain in their hands and feet due to nerve damage caused by diabetes. Goli studied 244 nondepressed diabetic patients who were randomly assigned to receive treatment for six weeks with either low-dose venlafaxine XR (75 mg/day), high-dose venlafaxine XR (150-225 mg/day), or a placebo (sugar pill). By the end of the study, 56 percent of patients receiving high-dose venlafaxine reported significantly less pain compared to 39 percent of patients receiving low-dose venlafaxine and 34 percent of those treated with placebo. In that study, nausea was the most commonly reported side effect (10 percent to 22 percent of those taking venlafaxine and 5 percent of those taking placebo). The reduced pain from treatment could not have been due to the treatment of depression, because patients with depression were excluded from the study.

Muscle Relaxants

Cyclobenzaprine (Flexeril) and methocarbamol (Robaxin) are medicines that help to relax tense muscles and thereby ease pain. Muscles may be tense because of psychological stress, a response to inflammation, or the body's response to pain itself. Whatever the cause, if muscles contract and tighten up, this reduces blood flow to the muscles—causing ischemia (lack of oxygen) that results in pain and inflammation. It is easy for a vicious cycle to develop, leading to more and more pain as muscles become more and more tense. Cyclobenzaprine and similar drugs help to interrupt this vicious cycle, increasing blood flow to muscles and reducing pain and inflammation. Sometimes very low doses of these medications are effective. For example, I have found that one-fourth of a 10 mg cyclobenzaprine at night helps to relieve my pain and keep me functional. Because my body will tend to get used to this small dose, I periodically need to give it a "drug holiday." This means doing without the drug for a week or ten days, allowing my body to become sensitive to it again.

Antianxiety Drugs

Diazepam (Valium) is the best known of the medications in this drug class, sometimes known as benzodiazepines. These medicines also serve to relax tense or spasmodic muscles, helping to break the vicious cycle of muscle contraction, ischemia, inflammation, and pain. Unfortunately, these drugs—especially the longer-acting ones—tend to accumulate in the body and result in oversedation, impaired concentration, poor reaction time, and problems with balance. These side effects are especially worrisome problems in persons aged sixty-five or older. Furthermore, the human body tends to quickly accommodate or get used to these drugs, requiring a person to take higher and higher doses to have the same effect when used chronically. Today, shorter-acting benzodiazepines exist that have fewer side effects and are therefore preferred (clonazepam or lorazepam, for example). Unless absolutely necessary, however, they should be avoided over the long term unless the person has a professionally diagnosed anxiety disorder.

Anticonvulsants

Because anticonvulsants help to calm irritable nerves, medicines such as phenytoin (Dilantin), carbamazepine (Tegretol), valproic acid (Depakote), and especially gabapentin (Neurontin) have been used effectively together with analgesics to treat chronic pain. Both tricyclic antidepressants and anticonvulsants reduce pain, especially neuropathic pain, by changing the characteristics of the nerve cell membrane by blocking "sodium channels."[15] Neuropathic pain syndromes include chronic pain following herpes zoster skin infection (postherpetic neuralgia), trigeminal neuralgia, and diabetic neuropathy. Apparently, pain from trauma (following injury or postsurgical syndromes) or from inflammatory disease (such as rheumatoid arthritis) doesn't respond as well. Lamotragine (Lamictal) is an anticonvulsant that may be particularly effective for lacinating or stabbing kinds of pain.

People with neuropathic pain who don't respond to one anticonvulsant may respond to another, so sometimes it takes some shopping around. Gabapentin (Neurontin) is perhaps the safest of the medicines noted since it has very few interactions with other drugs and does not affect the liver. This is not the case for phenytoin, carbamazepine, or valproic acid, which may either increase or decrease the metabolism (breakdown) of many other medicines, and may also have substantial side effects of their own. Gabapentin does not work for everyone, however. Furthermore, although 300 mg to 3,600 mg/day of this drug is usually effective, doses may need to be pushed up to 4,000 to

5,000 mg/day to maximize clinical benefit.[16] At those and even much lower doses, gabapentin may be associated with considerable sedation. The sedation tends to diminish over time with continued use of the drug. Gabapentin may be particularly effective for those with chronic pain who are irritable or angry, since studies have shown that anger scale scores diminish with the use of this medication.

Anticonvulsants are seldom used alone for the treatment of chronic pain, or as the drug of first choice; rather, they are usually used in association with other analgesics. However, the drug of first choice for treating neuropathic pain is a tricyclic antidepressant or venlafaxine (Effexor).[17] If neither of these is effective, then an anticonvulsant such as gabapentin may be tried. Combinations may also be useful in certain cases.

Topical Treatments

Topical agents are usually not very helpful because of the local irritation and, sometimes, allergic reactions they elicit. Topical treatments involve creams or ointments applied to the skin to either numb the skin or act as a counterirritant (distracting attention away from the pain site or possibly closing the "gate" in the spinal cord through which pain impulses must travel). Examples of counterirritants include capsaicin cream (made from hot chili peppers) or commercially available rubs (BenGay) that make the skin feel hot or cold. Examples of numbing agents include topical lidocaine or combinations of lidocaine and prilocaine. These are applied directly to the skin around the pain site as a cream or occlusive patch. Patches that deliver anti-inflammatory medication strictly to the pain site are also now being tested.[18]

Recommendation

Probably the safest and most effective drug treatment for persons with chronic pain, particularly that due to arthritis, is a combination of three drugs: acetaminophen, NSAIDs, and a muscle relaxant. They should first begin acetaminophen at a dose of 650 to 1,000 mg, scheduled regularly every six to eight hours (assuming the absence of liver disease, hypersensitivity to acetaminophen, or other contraindication). If pain is still not relieved and there is no history of gastrointestinal problems or hypersensitivity to NSAIDs, they should then begin a COX-2 inhibitor at a dose of 50 to 100 mg twice daily for celecoxib (unless there is a sulfa allergy) or 12.5 to 25 mg once daily for rofecoxib. If tolerated, the dose can be increased up to 200 mg twice daily of celecoxib or 25 mg twice daily of rofecoxib for time-limited periods. If pain persists, a low dose of muscle relaxant such as cyclobenzaprine 2.5 to 5.0 mg or a tricyclic antidepressant such as amitriptyline 10 to 25 mg should be added at bedtime. Sometimes a pain reliever used in combination with two antidepressants, such as 20 mg fluoxetine (Prozac) plus 25 mg amitriptyline (Elavil), is most effective. This regimen is not free of potential side effects, so regular monitoring for excessive sedation, gastrointestinal bleeding (by fecal occult blood tests), and kidney and liver problems, is necessary.

Summary

Most chronic pain can be controlled over the long term with nonnarcotic pain medication as described in this chapter. These, together with psychosocial, behavioral, spiritual, and nonsurgical mechanical treatments (discussed in Chapter 12), are usually sufficient to reduce pain to a tolerable level that enables function and a reasonable quality of life. Probably the best combination of drugs for chronic pain involves a pain reliever, an antidepressant, and if necessary, an anticonvulsant such as gabapentin. If these methods fail, however, and pain becomes intolerable, other pharmacologic strategies must be considered.

NARCOTIC ANALGESICS

Although their use is controversial in chronic pain states not caused by cancer, narcotic pain relievers do serve an important role in the treatment of chronic nonmalignant pain.[19] Concern regarding these drugs arises when they are used instead of a comprehensive pain management program. Narcotic pain relievers are easy to prescribe, easy and effortless to take, and are very effective in relieving pain. Careful monitoring, however, is necessary not only to prevent excessive use but also to treat the multiple side effects associated with long-term use of these drugs, such as constipation, difficulty concentrating, and excessive sedation, to name just a few.

Narcotic pain relievers are either derived naturally from the opium plant (such as morphine or codeine), or are synthesized in chemical laboratories (such as heroin, hydromorphone, or oxycodone). These drugs are typically used for the treatment of acute, severe, time-limited pain. Because the body tends to accommodate to these medicines when taken over long periods of time, doses may need to be increased to maintain the analgesic effect. For that reason and others, until recently opiates have been discouraged for the treatment of chronic pain that occurs outside a diagnosis of cancer or other terminal illnesses.

Aggressive use of narcotic analgesics for the treatment of pain from cancer or a terminal illness is now considered the standard of care. It is cruel to allow a patient with a terminal illness to suffer when effective pain treatments are readily available. Even the use of narcotic drugs for long-term noncancer pain, although controversial, is believed by some experts to be appropriate in certain circumstances, particularly elderly persons suffering from severe chronic pain.[20] A number of state agencies have now released guidelines for the use of narcotic pain relievers for noncancer related pain,[21] and federal guidelines also exist that specify the conditions under which prescribing narcotics for chronic pain is appropriate.[22] These experts maintain that concern about addiction, although still present, has been overemphasized in the past, depriving many sufferers of chronic pain much needed relief.[23] Says pain expert Dr. Dean Edell, "The risk of addiction for patients with no history of [alcohol or drug] abuse is minimal, according to recent studies, which show that less than one-half of one-percent of patients become addicted to their painkillers."[24]

Unfortunately, few studies have examined the effectiveness and duration of benefit when narcotic pain relievers are used to treat chronic noncancer pain. The American Academy of Pain Medicine and the American Pain Society have issued a joint statement concerning the use of opioids in the treatment of chronic pain.[25] Their recommendations follow.

First, they emphasize that chronic pain is common, affecting more than one-quarter of the American population, and that the economic cost is staggering, amounting to tens of billions of dollars annually. Second, they point out that many state boards of medical examiners have, due to ignorance, discouraged the use of opioids for chronic nonmalignant pain. Third, they indicate that chronic pain is often managed inadequately with nonopiate preparations. Fourth, they point out that the incidence of addiction in patients taking opioids for pain is low and there is generally no ceiling effect on analgesia (in other words, there is no dose above which no further pain relief can be obtained by increasing the dose, particularly for morphine). Tolerance to the drug's side effects usually develops; side effects such as sedation and nausea usually disappear with continued use; and constipation can be managed with diet, stool softeners, and laxatives. Fifth, although some opioids may be diverted to illegal sale or use, this should not prevent their use in the management of chronic pain. Finally, a single clinician should take primary responsibility for prescribing opioids for a patient with chronic pain.

A number of physiological studies support the use of opiates for chronic pain. For example, the effects of narcotic pain relievers in the body differ depending on whether the person is experiencing chronic pain or no pain.[26] Research has shown that the effect of narcotics on slowing the respiratory rate (speed of breathing) is reduced in subjects with pain compared to those without pain. When pain is experimentally reduced by performing a nerve block, any given dose of narcotic analgesic will have a greater effect on slowing the respiratory rate. This means that someone in true physical pain reacts differently to a narcotic drug than does someone without pain.

ADDICTION VERSUS PHYSICAL DEPENDENCE

It is important to distinguish addiction from physical dependence because these two terms are frequently confused. Addiction occurs when an individual seeks out a drug, has negative consequences resulting from use of the drug, and uses more and more of the drug than originally intended. Physical dependence occurs when a person has been taking a drug for a long time and his or her body becomes used to the drug. Discontinuing use of the drug after the body has grown used to it results in unpleasant physical symptoms (a withdrawal reaction). People with chronic pain may become physically dependent on either narcotic or nonnarcotic medications, so that when they stop the medication their pain gets worse and they also experience symptoms of drug withdrawal. Although addiction is associated with the need to take more and more medication to achieve the desired effect, people in chronic pain who are physically dependent on a medication sometimes need more medication because the pain at the lower dose was under-treated. These are not drug addicts but simply people with chronic pain who are dependent on the pain medication and need more of it for adequate pain relief.

Even many physicians do not truly understand the difference between addiction and physical dependence. The result is that physicians may fail to give adequate doses of pain medication for the amount of pain a person has. This is especially true for narcotic analgesics. Because this medication relieves the pain (as it relieved my pain from kidney stones), people in pain will want more of it. Doctors may then label these patients as addicts, which is simply not true—no more true than if a person with high blood pressure needed more high blood pressure medication because their disease, hypertension, was getting worse. Studies have shown that most doctors underprescribe medication for people in chronic pain.[27] They have also shown, however, that some doctors prescribe inappropriately large doses of pain medication. Either extreme results in poor management of chronic pain.

NARCOTIC PAIN RELIEVER OF FIRST CHOICE

Among opioids, the drug of first choice is morphine[28] (although this drug has traditionally not been given for nonmalignant chronic pain). To date, no other drug has a faster onset, longer effect, or better ratio of benefits to side effects. Speed of onset largely depends on the route of administration: the intravenous (IV) route has the fastest onset (two minutes), whereas sustained release oral preparations may take two to four hours to reach maximum effect. Intramuscular (IM) injection has a twenty-minute onset, and the usual oral preparations begin to work in about one hour. Speed of onset is relevant only when the drug is being taken on an as-needed or PRN basis; for patients needing continuous treatment, speed of onset is less important.

Morphine's major active metabolite (called M6G) is cleared by the kidneys, and dosage must be reduced for those with impaired renal function—especially for patients receiving a fixed dose of morphine on a regular schedule. Note also that renal function tends to decrease with age, requiring some dosage adjustment in the elderly.

Side Effects

Adverse side effects should be anticipated when using opioid drugs.[29] Persons taking these drugs should be monitored for excessive sedation, concentration problems, interference with driving, myoclonus (muscle jerks), and pruritis (itching). Side effects can be minimized by starting treatment with a low dose and slowly increasing it. Constipation is common and may be controlled by encouraging fluid intake and exercise, ensuring that impaction does not develop (hardened mass of stool that does not pass); osmotic, stimulant, or motility-enhancing laxatives may be used if necessary, whereas Metamucil-like agents should be avoided. Sedation and cognitive impairment can be particularly problematic for active people; such persons should avoid driving, be extra cautious to avoid falling or other accidents, and have a friend or family member monitor them for excess respiratory depression (less than eight breaths per minute). Nausea is one of the most unpleasant symptoms and often limits drug use, and may be handled by waiting for tolerance to develop, using antiemetics as necessary, or switching to different opioids, since not all of these drugs will produce the same degree of nausea. Itchiness can be intolerable, but may be controlled with antihistamines. Clonazepam can be used to treat myoclonus or muscle spasms (especially those occurring at night).

In a randomized study of forty-six patients with nonmalignant chronic pain who received oral morphine for a period of six weeks, only thirteen patients had dose-limiting adverse side effects. Of the forty-six patients, eighteen experienced nausea, seventeen dizziness, and nineteen constipation.[30] Thus, about 40 percent of patients had nausea or dizziness, to which tolerance developed relatively rapidly. The 40 percent of patients with constipation, however, did not readily develop tolerance to that side effect which had to be managed with increased fluids, exercise, and laxatives.

Opioid-Resistant Pain

Certain types of chronic noncancer pain (especially neuropathic pain) are not relieved by increasing doses of opioid analgesics. This is the kind of pain that Bob suffers (Chapter 3). Opioid-resistant pain is most often found in conditions in which nerves are either compressed or destroyed (following an accident or surgery), sometimes indicated by pain occurring in a numb area of the body. Some pain experts argue that the problem results from the inability to give a sufficiently high dose of narcotic pain reliever before the emergence of side effects that prevent further increases in dosage.[31] In that case, use of antidepressants, anticonvulsants, local anesthetics, or even spinal infusions (using mixtures of local anesthetic and opioids) may be necessary. Spinal infusions that combine a local anesthetic with an opioid enable use of relatively low doses of both medications, relieving pain before treatment-limiting side effects occur. The addition of the antihypertensive medication clonidine to the treatment regimen may provide further benefit for some people.[32]

COMBINING NARCOTIC
AND NONNARCOTIC ANALGESICS

Although careful monitoring is necessary to avoid drug interactions and side effects, people with chronic pain often benefit from combinations of narcotic and nonnarcotic analgesics. For example, aspirin or acetaminophen may be combined with small amounts of codeine resulting in better pain relief than if either drug were used alone. A recent study was done to see if patients receiving the NSAID naproxen (Naprosyn) for osteoarthritic knee pain could reduce their dose of naproxen if a synthetic narcotic analgesic called tramadol (Ultram) was added to the treatment regimen.[33] On average, subjects receiving 200 mg of tramadol per day were able to reduce their naproxen dose from 1,000 mg/day to 220 mg/day, compared to subjects receiving a placebo who could only reduce their naproxen dose to 410 mg/day. The investigators concluded that among patients with painful osteoarthritis of the knee responding to 1,000 mg per day of naproxen, the addition of tramadol 200 mg per day allowed a significant reduction in the dosage of naproxen with continued pain relief.

Algos Pharmaceutical Corporation has recently produced a new drug called MorphiDex that is a combination of morphine and an ingredient in cough medicine called dextromethorphan.[34] Preliminary research shows that due to its effects on nerve receptors, MorphiDex works about twice as fast and twice as long as morphine alone. This allows patients to take about half their usual dose of morphine, decreasing the likelihood of side effects. A number of strategies, then, may be tried when current treatment fails to provide pain relief or when drug side effects prohibit increases in dose.

MAXIMIZING EFFECTIVENESS OF MEDICATIONS

The purpose of pain medications is to reduce pain, increase physical functioning, and improve emotional distress and sleep. The schedule of medication dosing is very important. For patients with chronic, continuous pain, analgesics should be given regularly, not on an as-needed or PRN basis. Additional doses of medication may be given prior to performing particularly painful activities or exercising. A consensus panel of the American Geriatrics Society[35] makes the following summary recommendations for using medication to treat chronic pain:

- Fast onset, short-acting drugs should be used for episodic pain (pain that occurs now and then, but is not continuous).
- Acetaminophen should be used for mild to moderate pain (not exceeding 4,000 mg/day).
- NSAIDs should be tried next, but used with caution.
- Avoid high-dose, long-term NSAIDs if possible.
- If NSAIDs are used long term, try using on an as-needed or PRN basis rather than on a continuous basis to give the stomach and kidneys a break from exposure.
- Avoid NSAIDs in persons with kidney problems, a history of peptic ulcer disease, or bleeding tendency.
- Never use more than one NSAID type at a time (for example, aspirin and ibuprofen together).
- Consider opioid (narcotic) drugs for moderate to severe pain unrelieved by other pharmacologic and nonpharmacologic measures (especially for pain that has a clear physical cause, such as arthritis).
- Use long-acting or time-release opioid preparations (such as sustained-release morphine) for severe continuous pain.
- Use short-acting preparations with a fast onset (immediate-release morphine) for breakthrough pain (e.g., pain that suddenly worsens beyond the usual level).

- Increase the maintenance dose (e.g., regular daily dose) gradually and carefully, based on amount of medication used each day for breakthrough pain.
- Anticipate adverse effects of opioid drugs (as previously indicated).
- When using combinations of an opioid and acetaminophen or NSAID, be sure that the maximum safe dose of either acetaminophen or NSAID is not exceeded.
- Monitor those taking opioids for inappropriate, dangerous, or illicit drug use patterns (e.g., ask about prescriptions for pain medication from other doctors).
- Do not use opioids to treat anxiety or depression.
- If early refill requests for opioids are made, assess for development of tolerance, progression of disease, or illicit use.
- Monitor for gastrointestinal blood loss, kidney dysfunction, and drug/drug interactions.

RESEARCH ON NEW PAIN MEDICINES

Because there are so many people in America and around the world who experience chronic pain, drug companies are continuously looking for new medicines that are more effective and have fewer side effects.[36] According to the American Pain Society, nearly 45 percent of Americans will seek medical help for chronic pain at some time in their lives, with nearly 515 million workdays lost and 40 million doctor visits. The world market for pain relievers is about $8 billion and is growing at a rate of 7 percent per year.[37] Studies are being done to identify drugs that will bind to pain receptors in the spinal cord and brain, rather than just at the peripheral site of the pain. Other studies are looking at drugs that block pain-producing substances in the body such as "substance P." As noted earlier, drugs are being developed that show more and more specificity for the COX-2 enzyme, sparing the COX-1 enzyme.

New medicines now in the testing phase are called "smart drugs" because they are designed to go right to the site causing the pain (a painful joint, for example), but nowhere else in the body where they might cause side effects. Examples include Ziconotide and ABT-594. Ziconotide, produced by Neurex Corporation in Menlo Park, California, acts on the pain-sensitive nerves in the spinal cord, but not on other tissues in the body. ABT-594, produced by Abbott Laboratories in North Chicago, Illinois, acts on the same cellular mechanism as nicotine does in relieving anxiety; the result is a drug fifty times more potent than morphine.

New immune therapies are also under investigation for the treatment of autoimmune disorders such as rheumatoid arthritis and other types of inflammatory arthritis. A number of therapies target the key proinflammatory cytokines tumor necrosis factor (TNF) and interleukin-1 (IL-1). Two new inhibitors of TNF are the soluble TNF receptor construct etanercept (Enbrel) and the anti-TNF monoclonal antibody infliximab (Remicade by Centocor, Inc., Malvern, Pennsylvania). A recent double-blind placebo-controlled two-year trial with infliximab used along with methotrexate (MTX) found response rates in rheumatoid arthritis of 40 percent to 48 percent, compared to 16 percent in those taking MTX alone.[38] Similarly, a two-year study conducted at Stanford University used etanercept to treat aggressive rheumatoid arthritis, randomizing patients to receive either a rapidly increasing dose of MTX or 10 mg to 25 mg doses of etanercept twice weekly.[39] Both tolerability and clinical response to etanercept were greater than to MTX. Thus, within ten years we will no doubt see remarkable changes in the way chronic pain is treated.

NONDRUG TREATMENTS FOR PAIN

Nonpharmacological treatments should always be used along with drug therapy in the management of chronic pain, since these treatments may help to reduce the dose of medication needed for pain control. It should be emphasized here that attention to the nondrug aspects of therapy is at least as important if not more so, than medication. Nondrug treatments are discussed in greater detail in Chapters 10, 11, 12, and 15.

First, there is education—education about the pain, education about the drugs used to treat the pain, and education about other ways of relieving the pain besides medication. Both the person in pain *and* his or her family or caregiver need such education.

Second, cognitive-behavioral therapy might relieve the depression and anxiety that go hand in hand with chronic pain. Altering beliefs, attitudes, and thoughts about pain often helps to relieve the suffering that pain causes. Biofeedback, progressive relaxation, meditation, and prayer can also be used effectively to reduce the intensity of the pain or to help a person to cope better with it. These approaches have no side effects and provide those in chronic pain with tools to help themselves.

Third, physical or occupational therapy should always be included to increase joint range of motion and to reduce muscle weakness. This includes instruction on how to begin an exercise program to keep weight down, increase flexibility, and maintain conditioning. Exercise also makes people feel better about themselves and helps relieve some of the side effects seen with medications (e.g., constipation). However, it is important to carefully balance physical activity with rest; otherwise, muscles or joints may be strained and pain may worsen.

Fourth, transcutaneous electrical nerve stimulation (TENS) may be very effective even when pain medications are not. TENS units are particularly helpful for persons with chronic low back pain or other types of neuropathic pain that results from compression or crush injury to nerves. Use of heat or cold packs may likewise be helpful, but it is important to avoid thermal injury to the skin that often follows prolonged applications. All of these areas will be addressed in greater depth in other chapters.

SUMMARY AND CONCLUSIONS

Treatment approaches for acute and chronic pain differ. In acute, time-limited pain, every effort should be made to provide comfort with rapid-acting pain relievers. The same is true for pain that occurs in the setting of terminal illness. With chronic pain, drug treatment should be accompanied by rehabilitation that reduces the psychological consequences of pain, increases function, and enhances quality of life. Drug treatments for chronic pain should begin with medications that have the fewest side effects (acetaminophen, NSAIDs, muscle relaxants, antidepressants) and proceed as necessary to those with more long-term consequences (narcotic pain relievers).

Although most persons with mild to moderate pain will receive adequate relief with nonnarcotic analgesics, some persons with severe chronic pain will require opiates to maintain function and some degree of quality life. Combinations of narcotic and nonnarcotic medications are sometimes more effective than either alone. Regardless of the specific type of drug, side effects should be anticipated and treated prophylactically. New scientific advances will soon provide us with medications that are capable of relieving pain more effectively with fewer side effects. Nondrug therapies should be used alongside of medications to help minimize the drug doses required for pain relief and the suffering that pain causes.

Chapter 10

Psychosocial and Behavioral Treatments

Psychological and social factors have an enormous influence on the experience of pain, and vice versa. Therapies have been developed to address these psychosocial factors and thereby relieve some of the suffering that accompanies chronic pain. Depression, anxiety, loneliness, feelings of abandonment, and loss of control often greatly magnify the intensity of pain—or at least its perceived intensity. There are also a number of psychological and social consequences of chronic pain itself, including depression, personality changes, insomnia, fatigue, weight problems, decreased ability to get about and care for oneself, problems with social relationships, and family problems. A common reaction to pain is frustration, irritability, and anger. The frequency of these emotional responses increases as the duration of pain increases. They are heavily influenced by an individual's underlying personality. Before discussing therapies, however, some of these psychosocial and behavioral problems are described in greater detail.

PSYCHOSOCIAL AND BEHAVIORAL CONSEQUENCES OF CHRONIC PAIN

Depression

There is a strong positive correlation between depression and pain—sometimes so strong that the two are difficult to tell apart. In a review of 191 separate studies of the depression/chronic pain relationship as part of a workshop sponsored by the National Institutes of Health, researchers reported there was a consistent relationship between chronic pain and depression.[1] They concluded that chronic pain is more likely to cause depression, than depression is to cause chronic pain.

As noted earlier, however, depression may worsen the perceived severity of pain.

Among those with chronic pain, it is also not uncommon to find suicidal thoughts, and failed and successful suicide attempts increase with the duration of pain.[2] This is not surprising given that serious depression occurs in nearly one-half of all chronic pain sufferers.[3] People often have difficulty separating emotional from physical pain (as do doctors). The disability and life changes brought on by chronic pain involve tremendous loss and grief over that loss. As emotional pain worsens, the person tends to focus more on the pain and think more negatively about it, which magnifies the pain and further increases suffering, plunging the person into a downward spiral.

A former patient of mine, Jane, was suffering from chronic low back pain following spinal surgery. She was depressed and discouraged over the failed operation and the changes the pain had caused in her life. She was forced to retire from an exciting job that had given her life meaning and purpose, and was now also experiencing significant financial strain. She had lost interest in and stopped doing many of the activities that she still could do due to her depression. She spent much of her time at home ruminating about her pain and inability to work. She stopped exercising and began to gain weight, which further exacerbated her pain. She lost interest in sex, and even emotional intimacy became difficult as her irritability and decreasing self-esteem began to affect her relationship with her husband. This case, however, had a good outcome. With antidepressant medication and psychotherapy, her spirits lifted and her pain became more tolerable, and her activities increased. As she began to feel better about herself, her relationships with her husband and family improved.

Suffering

Chapman and Gavrin distinguish suffering from depression by noting that suffering is a "broader, more inclusive concept than depression; not necessarily a psychopathological state; not necessarily associated with self blame or self-deprecation; and more dependent on awareness of the future" (p. 2234).[4]

How is suffering related to pain? Pain in its purest form is a disturbing physical sensation that results from damage to nerve tissue or alterations in the nervous system from previous damage. Suffering involves both these disturbing physical sensations and the ongoing effect that conscious awareness of physical pain has on the psychological self. To better understand this second component of suffering, it is necessary to examine the different aspects of the self that have been identified. In the brain, a coherent map of the physical body is maintained called the "physical self " or "body self." When a person loses an arm in an accident, the representation of the arm in the brain remains intact, giving rise to phantom limb sensations (pain perceived in an arm no longer present).

Composing the psychological self are an "agent self," a "cognitive self," and a "dynamic self."[5] The agent self is goal oriented and helps to define a social identity by interacting with others in an attempt to fulfill its needs. The cognitive self is how one thinks about oneself and is based on the individual's history and future (i.e., personal story). The dynamic self is viewed as a changing entity that emerges through the life course, being based first largely on physical attributes but later on wisdom, inward growth, and relationships with others.

It is important to understand how physical pain can affect these different aspects of the self and thereby result in suffering. Pain involves the physical sensation of damage to the physical body (body self) and the emotional reaction to that threat to biological survival. Suffering, as noted previously, is a much broader psychological and social phenomenon than is physical pain. These other elements involve a perception of threat to the psychological self in terms of loss of self-esteem, role in family and community, and purpose in life.

The extent to which severe, prolonged pain will result in changes to the psychological self is largely dependent on the particular function impacted most by the pain. For example, if painful arthritis in her ankles interferes with a young professional skater's ability to continue in her profession (on which her cognitive and dynamic images of self are at least partially based), then this will create suffering of much greater magnitude than would ankle arthritis for an older retired person. For the older retired person, however, this might interfere with socialization and defining relationships, thereby also causing a threat to the agent self and resulting in suffering from unmet social needs (loneliness).

Pain can result in a loss of control over one's circumstances or environment, creating dependency on others that may be very stressful for someone whose cognitive self is rooted in their independence and self-sufficiency. The dysfunction caused by pain can give rise to negative cognitions (thinking pessimistically that the pain will never improve, that it is incompatible with a fulfilling life) or dysfunctional beliefs (that pain will result in severe disability or an agonizing death) which further act as stressors.

The resulting psychological stress can activate the hypothalamic-pituitary axis increasing autonomic nervous system activity and the release of stress hormones (cortisol, epinephrine, etc.) that ultimately interfere with immune and cardiovascular systems, which may be depended on for healing the physical condition responsible for the pain. Chronic pain, then, commonly results in a host of problems including chronic fatigue, insomnia, social withdrawal, and impaired immune and neuroendocrine functioning that can worsen physical and mental performance—leading to a self-perpetuating cycle of stress, disability, and dependency.

Chronic pain affects one's productivity in all aspects of life, including work, home, and the wider social environment. The person can no longer do the things that he or she once did which gave life purpose, and he or she fears this will continue indefinitely. This discrepancy among the past, present, and future images of the self is the essence of suffering and results from damage to the integrity of the self.[6] As this discrepancy becomes wider, a loss of hope begins to creep in —hope that the person will ever return to doing the things that defined who he or she was, that gave life meaning. This leads to depression.

Understanding how pain results in suffering will help caretakers more effectively relieve suffering. The meaning of the pain to the individual and its impact on self-image is particularly important. Because uncontrolled physical pain prevents people from doing things that define who they are, every effort should be made to provide pain relief. By relieving the physical pain, the person not only feels better but also functions better, thus helping to avoid some of the changes in the psychological self that lie at the root of both depression and suffering.

Anxiety

Anxiety and fear are strongly associated with pain, particularly as pain increases in severity. Pain increases anxiety because the person worries that the pain will never end. A sense of control is lost and feelings of helplessness ensue. Anxiety results in muscle tension and spasm, reducing blood flow and increasing tissue ischemia, releasing chemicals into the surrounding tissues that worsen the physical pain, and on the cycle goes. By addressing these fears about the person's current and future life, some psychological relief can be provided even if the physical pain cannot be eliminated.

This was the situation with Henry, who came to see me after experiencing worsening anxiety and panic attacks following the development of chronic pain from advancing rheumatoid arthritis. Henry's pain medications were no longer working, he said, and he was experiencing neck and back spasms in addition to his swollen joints. Despite being on maximum therapy for his arthritis, he felt his pain increasing and there was nothing he could do to stop it. He was becoming increasingly irritable and anxious. Further history revealed problems in his family, and that his wife, on whom he was quite dependent, was threatening to leave him. Antianxiety medications and marital therapy were key factors in helping to relieve Henry's anxiety and to increase his support in the home, which subsequently improved his pain control.

Sleep Problems

Problems sleeping are often the most disabling consequence of chronic pain.[7] Restless, disturbed sleep becomes more and more common as the duration of the pain increases. In surveys of people experiencing pain from back problems, fibromyalgia, and rheumatoid arthritis, between 50 percent and 80 percent complain of sleep disturbance.[8] The sleep of those with chronic pain is often light, easily disrupted, and poorly restorative. The person typically wakes up tired with musculoskeletal stiffness and greater sensitivity to pain. A lack of restorative sleep contributes further to a downward plunge resulting from increased sensitivity to pain, depression, disrupted sleep, and so on.

Researchers evaluated the quality of sleep in 105 consecutive patients seen in a multidisciplinary chronic pain clinic.[9] Nearly two-thirds (65 percent) complained of poor sleep. Both sleep onset and sleep maintenance were disturbed in 67 percent and 74 percent of patients, respectively. In 85 percent of cases, sleep problems began at the same time or after the pain began. Cognitive-behavioral interventions that address negative thoughts about pain and self (as previously discussed) may improve sleep.[10]

Loss of Control

Treatments designed to give people a sense of control over their pain can often lead to improved coping and less impairment. Dr. Amy S. Badura of Creighton University in Omaha, Nebraska, and her colleagues surveyed seventy-three patients about their beliefs regarding control of their pain before and after a forty-hour, four-week outpatient pain management program.[11] Those who believed that control over the pain existed within themselves (rather than with some outside force such as fate, luck, or chance) coped significantly better, were less impaired, and had overall better functioning. Note that depending on God as an agent of control is actually a form of internal control, because prayer empowers individuals by giving them a tool to affect their own situation, rather than standing by helplessly or relying on others (more on this in Chapter 14).

Socialization

As noted earlier, chronic pain often causes social isolation and intense loneliness. Some people with chronic pain feel as though no one in the world can truly understand them (recall the words of Bob and Laura in Chapters 3 and 5). They may be irritable and rejecting of others, often a result of low self-esteem and defensiveness against fear that others will reject them. These persons need support and encouragement from others on a regular and persistent basis. Research has shown that even a simple monthly telephone call can result in significant improvement in pain and ability to function.

People with chronic pain also need to be encouraged to become involved in social activities, overcoming the initial resistance to such involvement. Even more important, they should be encouraged to provide support—particularly spiritual support—to others with similar problems. Such other-directed activities have repeatedly been shown to increase well-being, improve quality of life, and reduce depression.[12,13]

Behavioral Changes

Chronic pain often forces a reduction in physical activity, resulting in deconditioning, weak muscles, loss of flexibility, and disturbances in walking and balance. Because activities that used to provide pleasure can no longer be accomplished, the person's world becomes severely constricted. Eating is often one of the last pleasures to remain, and results in weight gain and further stress on joints, which increases pain and restricts activity. Deconditioning and weight changes also impact a person's self-esteem, adversely affecting socialization and leading to isolation and loneliness. The person begins to dwell more on pain and poor quality of life, thereby reinforcing the downward trajectory of decline and dysfunction.

In summary, pain causes psychological, social, and behavioral changes that adversely affect self-image and radically impair quality of life. Those changes, in turn, influence the perceived severity of pain and magnify the disability and dysfunction it causes. Psychosocial and behavioral therapies, then, provide tools for breaking this vicious cycle.

TREATMENTS FOR PSYCHOSOCIAL AND BEHAVIORAL PROBLEMS

Psychological

Psychological treatments seek to change a person's thoughts, beliefs, and attitudes toward pain. If everything that can be done biologically for pain has been done, then one must start dealing with it psychologically. Understandably, most persons resist pain and try desperately to escape it. However, other approaches may be more effective. One involves transforming the meaning of the pain. Another involves accepting the pain and moving on with life despite the pain.

Still another seeks to focus on the good that can result from (and *is* resulting from) the pain. Each of these changes in perspective and attitude is a goal of cognitive therapy.

Cognitive-behavioral therapy (CBT) is a common and widely used psychological treatment for pain in which the individual learns to think and behave in a healthy way that improves his or her outlook. CBT is designed to alter a patient's negative, pessimistic thought patterns and to engage him or her in behaviors that will improve mood and reduce pain. This frequently involves education, monitoring of thoughts and behaviors, rehearsal and initiation of new healthy patterns, and careful attention over time to maintain those healthy thoughts and behaviors.

Examples of commonly held catastrophic, excessively pessimistic thoughts about pain include: "My pain is intolerable," "I can't stand this pain any longer," "The pain will get so bad that I will go crazy," "This pain is uncontrollable," "The pain is destroying my life," "I can't live life in this kind of pain," "The pain will never get any better," and so forth. These negative thoughts, often not based in reality, lead to painful emotions, fear, and suffering. CBT helps people to recognize these thoughts and their relationship to emotions, helps them to consciously stop such negative thinking habits, and teaches them to counteract negative thoughts with healthy, reality-based positive thinking.

Objective research has verified the usefulness of CBT in the treatment of chronic pain. For example, researchers conducted a clinical trial to evaluate the effectiveness of CBT compared with standard treatment alone in the management of patients with chronic pain from rheumatoid arthritis.[14] A total of thirty-nine patients, three-quarters of them women, who averaged fifty-three years of age were randomized to either CBT ($n = 19$) or a control group ($n = 20$). Medication use was carefully monitored to ensure that both groups received equal medical treatment. The group receiving CBT had twelve weekly ninety-minute sessions of cognitive therapy that focused on helping patients to deal better with their pain. Patients were first educated about the gate-control theory of pain and the cycle of pain, muscle tension, and depression. Then CBT was described, including how it worked. Subjects were instructed to keep diaries on their negative, maladaptive thinking ("catastrophizing," helplessness, etc.), and encouraged to replace this type of thinking with more rational, reality-based thoughts and behaviors. Distraction techniques were encouraged, and patients were trained to focus their attention on pleasant activities. In particular, activity goals were scheduled and performance of enjoyable activities was reinforced at each session.

After three months of treatment, patients who received CBT experienced a 29 percent reduction in pain (a significant 18 percent greater than the control group). Neither group showed increases in measures of inflammation during the twelve-week study, as would be expected with this chronic progressive rheumatological disease. However, the CBT group experienced a significantly greater reduction in depression, anxiety, and helplessness compared to the control group. There was also an increase in positive thinking and positive acceptance in the CBT group. The significant amount of pain reduction possible through psychological interventions (18 percent in this study) is consistent with what other studies have reported.[15] Apart from pain intensity, this study also found significant effects for CBT on actual functioning, suggesting that pain was causing less disability in those who received the therapy.

In one of the largest studies examining the benefits of CBT for chronic pain, researchers observed 170 patients with severe chronic pain who completed a ten-week course of therapy.[16] At the end of the treatment, self-efficacy (measured by the ability to independently manage pain and to cope despite persistent pain) had improved by 31 percent. Pain intensity declined by 23 percent, disability by 19 percent, and depression by 27 percent. After one year, improvement in self-efficacy persisted while pain intensity, disability, and depression all continued to improve in the forty-one patients who completed the follow-up survey. By one year following treatment, pain intensity had decreased overall by 27 percent, disability by 36 percent, and depression by 41 percent. These differences remained significant even after controlling for differences in pain intensity, use of antidepressants, and use of narcotic pain relievers.

A spiritual form of CBT is described in an easy-to-read book called *Telling Yourself the Truth.*[17] Although this book does not specifically focus on pain, the principles discussed completely apply to those battling chronic pain. Spiritual CBT helps the person to conform their thinking pattern to the truth of biblical Scripture, not to the false foundations of fear, worry, and hopelessness.

Social Support

A number of studies have shown that increasing social support may help to reduce the suffering associated with chronic pain and may also increase physical functioning. For example, in a randomized clinical trial involving fifty-three patients with rheumatoid arthritis, an intervention involving psychological treatment and social support resulted in improved pain behavior, reduced anxiety, and even less disease activity when measured immediately following treatment and then again six months later.[18] The social support program was particularly helpful for relieving anxiety. In another study, investigators examined the effects of family support on treatment outcome in 181 persons participating in an outpatient chronic pain program. In this study, those with nonsupportive families tended to use more medication, reported more pain, and had lower activity levels than those with supportive families.[19]

In yet another study, investigators followed forty persons with osteoarthritis for one year, assessing joint pain and physical functioning.[20] Subjects either received an intervention that involved laypersons calling subjects on the telephone every month or were assigned to a control group. Persons with chronic pain from arthritis who received the telephone calls reported significantly less pain ($p < .01$) and also tended to show better physical functioning than those in the control group. This study is particularly important because it shows how community groups, such as religious organizations, could help people with chronic pain, e.g., by mobilizing lay volunteers to provide supportive contacts during the week.

The establishment of a support group for persons with chronic pain is an excellent way to reduce isolation and to increase socialization. A support group occurs when people with similar problems come together to talk, support each other, and share common experiences. For the person in chronic pain, a support group is a place to meet people who struggle as they do. One cannot fully understand what it's like to be in constant pain unless one has had the experience. In addition to receiving emotional support, members receive up-to-date information regarding the newest treatments for pain through newsletters and contact with other people coping daily with pain. As people share their burdens and sufferings with each other, there comes greater understanding, a sense of belonging, and a reduction in loneliness.

In Chapter 3, Bob experienced an improvement in his ability to cope with his pain when he formed a support group with other pain sufferers. This helped enormously to combat the social isolation that he felt from friends, family, and other church members, whom he believed could not truly understand what it was like to be in constant pain.

Behavioral Therapies

In the 1960s, now world-renowned scientist Ron Melzack at McGill University developed a theory to explain the physiological mechanism by which psychological and social factors might influence pain (the gate-control theory of pain).[21] He noticed that pain intensity appeared to be affected by attention, anxiety, suggestion, and other psychological and social influences. Melzack proposed that pain signals from an injured part of the body were influenced at the spinal cord level by nerve messages coming from other areas of the body and, especially, by nerve messages coming from the brain. His theory stated that a mechanism existed in the dorsal part of the spinal cord that acted as a gate to either inhibit or facilitate transmission of pain impulses. The function of this gate was dependent on simultaneous nerve inputs from both peripheral body sources and from the brain. He proposed that psychological influences, including past experience, attention, and other cognitive functions and behaviors, could inhibit pain transmission by closing the gate. This work became the scientific rationale underlying behavioral treatments for chronic pain during the past three decades.

There have been vigorous efforts to develop psychological and behavioral treatments for chronic pain during the past three decades. Among these treatments are hypnosis, biofeedback, relaxation training, meditation, and a variety of distraction techniques. These behavioral methods reduce helplessness and loss of control by providing practical tools that can be used to gain control over pain (which is of crucial importance) and reduce the need for medication. A number of studies have now shown that these techniques can be effective for reducing pain intensity.[22-24]

Visualization and Relaxation

Visualization and progressive relaxation can help to reduce muscle tension contributing to pain. The person is taught to visualize himself or herself in a beautiful and relaxed natural setting (sitting on the grass next to a calm, serene mountain lake; lying on the beach by the ocean; or sitting on a cool rock in the middle of a valley stream in springtime).

Progressive muscle relaxation is often combined with visualization to help induce a state of deep relaxation and decreased pain. The person learns to consciously tense muscles for ten seconds and then relax them, beginning with the muscles of the forehead and then slowly going down the body to the muscles of the face, neck, chest, back, arms, torso, upper legs, lower legs, and feet. Each muscle group is tensed and then fully and completely relaxed, often while saying to oneself, "I am feeling more relaxed, more peaceful, more comfortable, and totally at ease."

Dr. Herbert Benson, from Harvard Medical School, discovered a physiological response that he called the relaxation response.[25] Many different methods may be used to induce the relaxation response, including both Eastern meditation and Judeo-Christian prayer. The usual procedure is to clear the mind of miscellaneous thoughts, monitor breathing, and focus on a word or phrase which is repeated over and over again. This technique has been shown to evoke a state of deep relaxation that reduces pain and anxiety and produces other positive mental and physiological changes.

Biofeedback and Hypnosis

Biofeedback is a process in which the patient is provided with visual or auditory feedback on physiological functioning and level of relaxation. This facilitates the learning of self-control over pain. By having immediate visual feedback, this helps the person to learn to relax and thereby lower pain intensity. A variety of machines provide the visual feedback required for such learning.

An electromyogram (EMG) records the tension or level of contraction of a muscle or muscle group; this level of tension is then displayed on a monitor screen to provide immediate feedback to the patient about his or her level of relaxation. An electroencephalogram (EEG) involves placing electrical leads onto the scalp to detect small electrical impulses given off by the brain, called brain waves; by displaying the brain waves on a computer monitor that the patient observes, immediate feedback is provided on whether thoughts and emotions are either stressed or relaxed. A skin conductance amplifier (SCA) measures the skin's ability to conduct electricity. Skin conductance depends on the amount of moisture or perspiration emitted by the skin. Perspiration facilitates the flow of electricity and is dependent on the emotional and physical state of the individual. Pulse rate and blood pressure can also be measured and displayed upon a screen to provide immediate feedback about a person's level of stress or pain.

Hypnosis is a technique whereby the patient is trained to enter into a state of deep relaxation and concentrated attention to consciously decrease concentration on pain sensations. Some may view hypnosis as a New Age spiritual technique that involves loss of control of one's body or mind to the influence of another person. Although hypnosis may be used for negative or destructive purposes (as can any other healing technique), it can also be used for good. Learning self-hypnosis can help the person with chronic pain to distract his or her attention away from the pain without fear of being unduly influenced by others. When employed appropriately and skillfully, hypnosis has been used to successfully reduce pain during dental procedures, some types of surgery, and even childbirth without the use of pain medication.

Laughter

Scripture says, "A cheerful heart is good medicine, but a crushed spirit dries up the bones" (Proverbs 17:22). Indeed, at least a couple of studies indicate that laughter may be an antidote for mild pain. In one study, researchers experimentally induced pain in twenty male and twenty female subjects. Pain was reported to be less severe in subjects listening to a twenty-minute comedy tape, compared to those listening to a dull narrative tape or no tape at all. Laughter, but not simple distraction, was found to alter the pain threshold.[26]

Likewise, in a study of ten healthy male volunteers, five subjects watched a sixty-minute humorous video and five subjects did not. Serial measurements were made of serum adrenocorticotropic hormone, cortisol, beta-endorphin, and 3,4-dihydroxyphenylacetic acid (or DOPAC, the major metabolite of dopamine, epinephrine, norepinephrine, growth hormone, and prolactin). Both cortisol and DOPAC showed significant decreases from baseline level in those watching the humor video compared to the control group. Furthermore, growth hormone levels in the experimental group significantly increased during baseline and decreased with the laughter intervention. Investigators concluded that laughter appeared to reduce serum levels of cortisol, DOPAC, epinephrine, and growth hormone, all indicating positive and healthy physiological responses.[27]

MULTIDISCIPLINARY TEAM APPROACH

In most cases, chronic pain cannot be cured or completely eliminated. This means that people need to learn to cope with the multiple physical, psychological, and social changes caused by pain. A multidisciplinary team approach is absolutely essential to help the person address these changes over the long term. The goal of treatment is to reduce the pain as much as possible and reinvolve the person in life.

SUMMARY AND CONCLUSIONS

Chronic pain often results in psychological, emotional, and social problems. Depression, anxiety, loss of control, loneliness, and social isolation are widespread. These problems, in turn, worsen the severity of the pain and are largely responsible for the suffering that accompanies pain. Professional therapies have been developed to help combat the negative thought processes and behaviors caused by chronic pain.

Cognitive therapy helps to encourage optimistic, reality-based thinking that leads to positive emotions and helps to discourage pessimistic, catastrophic thinking that leads to negative emotions. Social therapies strengthen social bonds in the family and community, combat loneliness, and reduce social isolation. Involvement in support groups made up of others with chronic pain is another effective method for achieving these ends. Behavioral therapies take advantage of the mind/body relationship and gate-control theory of pain and help to increase activity and develop self-control over pain. Humor and laughter can also help to reduce the suffering associated with pain. The effective management of chronic pain requires a multidisciplinary approach to attack the pain from many different angles and areas of expertise.

Chapter 11

Alternative and Complementary Treatments

"Natural" or "organic" treatments for pain can be acquired in health food stores, vitamin outlets, via the Internet, or through private individuals operating out of their homes, and they are available without prescription. These treatments offer an attractive alternative to expensive prescription pain medications with unpleasant and possibly dangerous side effects. Complementary and alternative medicine (CAM) is a huge industry—with over 42 percent of the U.S. population using alternative therapies.[1] These treatments are used to relieve pain from back injury, arthritis, and fibromyalgia. Nearly 70 percent of patients with cancer seek alternative therapies for treatment and pain relief.

Eisenberg and colleagues estimated that the out-of-pocket expenditures relating to alternative therapies were $27 billion in 1997, which is comparable to the out-of-pocket expenditures for *all* U.S. physician services.[2] Consequently, every charlatan has gone into the business hoping to make a profit. Even many hospitals are getting involved to increase their profit margin and assure their own survival in a perilous health care market.

This chapter reviews various types of alternative or complementary treatments for chronic pain, including herbal medicines and alternative procedures (acupuncture, use of magnets, etc.). Some of these treatments help to relieve pain, and do so with a minimum of cost or side effects. Others increase hope of relief, but don't deliver. Instead they often drain the bank accounts of desperate people ready to try anything. Many unproven natural therapies are no more effective than taking a sugar pill or other inactive ingredient. The mind is so powerful that it can either increase the pain threshold or lower it (whether or not the treatment helps). The more strongly a person believes in the treatment, the more likely it will work.

Many of these compounds and procedures have never been studied, so we simply don't know if they are effective. Even if a substance is found ineffective in general, however, it may be effective for a particular person. Each person's physiology or biological makeup is different. In an individual case, then, it is difficult to predict whether a treatment will or will not work, even for treatments proven scientifically to be effective. So there is always hope that one of these alternative treatments might work for an individual. That hope, however, should be a sensible one.

Whatever alternative medical treatments are chosen to relieve chronic pain, it is important that the person's doctor knows about them and that he or she integrates those treatments into the overall treatment plan. Although physicians may or may not agree with the choice to use alternative treatments, they will appreciate their patients' willingness to share this information with them. In the old days, the physician dictated what the patient would do and the patient complied. Today, that is no longer the case. Physician and patient must work together as members of a treatment team whose goals are to maximize pain relief, improve quality of life, and increase ability to function.

HERBAL MEDICINES

Herbal medicines taken for chronic pain should be used cautiously. The plant material being promoted as an herbal remedy may contain hundreds of different compounds. Only one or two of those compounds may be effective for treating pain. Does every plant have the same level of these pain-relieving compounds? When a company makes capsules or pills from this plant, does it measure the active ingredients or simply measure the weight of the leaves, stems, or root? This doesn't mean that herbal compounds don't work or aren't effective in relieving pain, only that buyers need to be sure of what they're getting and how much.

Isn't there a government agency that helps to protect the consumer from bad products sold in health food stores? Unfortunately, there is not. A federal act in 1994 removed vitamins, dietary supplements, herbs, and natural products from Food and Drug Administration (FDA) control. The FDA now has to prove that the product is bad before the product can be removed from the market. There is no regulation of purity, shelf life, or standardization, and no mandatory reporting of dangerous side effects. According to *Forbes Magazine,* this act by the federal government should be known as the "Food Fraud Facilitation Act."[3] For example, an analysis of the results of fifty preparations of ginseng sold in health food stores found problems of purity, contamination, and undeclared pharmaceuticals in one-third of these preparations.[4]

Taking a pill is fast and easy. It requires very little effort or exertion, which is why alternative therapies and herbal preparations are so attractive, especially in a culture where the quick fix is preferred over more long-term solutions. However, this may not be the most effective treatment for many pain conditions, especially conditions such as arthritis. Having hope in a pill can distract the person from engaging in activities proven to make a difference, such as weight loss, proper nutrition, and exercise. These all require effort and discipline, but promise real long-term benefits in terms of pain relief and prevention of pain-related complications. With these warnings in mind, descriptions of a number of herbal preparations that have been marketed as pain relievers are discussed next.

Herbal Preparations for Pain

Kava (Piper methysticum)

Kava is a flowering shrub that grows naturally in the South Pacific. The roots are used to prepare a drink (called kava-kava) that is used to treat migraine headache, gout, rheumatic conditions, menstrual cramps, anxiety, and insomnia. Kava is also available as a capsule, liquid extract, powder, and dried root. The active ingredient is kavalactone, which has been shown in animal studies to reduce glutamate levels in the brain (glutamate is an excitatory neurotransmitter associated with anxiety and agitation). Several studies in humans have found kava more effective than placebo in reducing anxiety. However, it does have a number of side effects including balance problems, double vision, excessive sedation, and liver dysfunction. Kava may also potentiate the effects of alcohol or other sedatives, and be associated with a dry, scaly, widespread dermatitis; it may be contraindicated in combination with benzodiazepines.

A typical kava drink contains about 250 milligrams (mg) of kavalactones. During social events among South Pacific natives, several drinks may be consumed at a time. A 250 mg capsule of the extract typically contains 75 mg of kavalactones. Approximately 24 to 70 mg kavalactones taken three times per day is reported to have a calming effect, and a dose of 180 to 210 mg kavalactones may be taken at bedtime to relieve insomnia. Research does exist demonstrating effects on reducing anxiety,[5] although no studies on pain exist. Safety is not proven and potency of commercial preparations may vary widely.

Japanese Mint (Mentha arvensis *var.* piperascens)

As a skin rub, Japanese mint is used for muscle and nerve pain. In Asia, it is used to treat joint pain and headache. As a member of the mint family, it is a source of menthol, a common ingredient in ointments such as ArthriCare or Eucalyptamint. It has a cooling effect on the skin that may distract attention away from the underlying site of pain. Japanese mint should not be taken internally by those who have a blocked bile duct, gallbladder inflammation, or severe liver damage. Japanese mint oil is available in oily and semisolid preparations. For internal use, advocates recommend placing two drops of the oil into a glass of water, tea, or juice, which is taken once or twice daily. No more than six drops per day of the oil is recommended. For external use, rub a few drops on the affected area. Overdose can occur, since the ingestion of as little as 2 grams of menthol may be fatal.

White Willow (Salix *spp.*)

Also known as European willow or salicin willow, this substance has been used for pain and rheumatism for nearly 2,000 years and may be the original source of aspirin. The white willow is a tree native to Central and Southern Europe and grows to a height of 20 to 50 feet. The active ingredient lies in the bark. Stomach problems are its primary side effect. White willow should not be taken if an aspirin allergy is present. To prepare a tea for internal consumption, put 2 to 3 grams (about 1¼ to 2 teaspoonfuls) of cut or coarsely powdered white willow in cold water, bring to a boil, steep for 5 minutes, then strain. The average daily dose that some recommend is 60 to 120 mg of the active ingredient salicin, or one cup of tea three to five times a day. Safety is not proven and potency of commercial preparations may vary widely.

Arnica (Arnica montana)

Arnica consists of the dried flower heads of *Arnica montana* or other *Arnica* species, which have bright yellow flowers reminiscent of daisies. The underground roots of the plant are sometimes utilized as well. Arnica is used as a general counterirritant, anti-inflammatory, and pain reliever. Arnica formulations may be rubbed into swollen ankles, dislocated shoulders, aching muscles, or arthritic joints. It is available as a liquid for compresses and poultices, an ointment, or a tincture. Arnica-containing creams are popular in Europe. A compress is made using one tablespoon tincture per half-liter water. For use in poultices, the tincture is diluted three to ten times with water. The ointment is used in maximum concentrations of 15 percent arnica oil or 20 to 25 percent tincture. Do not use arnica internally or on broken skin. Safety is not proven and potency of commercial preparations may vary widely.

Camphor (Cinnamomum camphora)

Camphor is obtained by steam distilling the parts of a tall flowering east Asian tree called *Cinnamomum camphora*. Camphor is typically used in the form of an oil. Camphor can be found in many topical medications to cool and soothe muscle aches and pains and reduce pain from inflamed arthritic joints. Camphor is for external use only and is available as a gel, drops, oil, ointment, or other formulation for use on the skin. In the United States, commercial topical preparations contain concentrations of up to 11 percent camphor and should be applied no more than four times per day. Safety is not proven and potency of commercial preparations may vary widely.

Oil of Wintergreen

This is one of the oldest treatments for pain. Derived from wintergreen shrubs, the active ingredient in the leaves of this plant is methyl salicylate, closely related to aspirin. The same product can be obtained from the bark of the cherry birch. Today the substance is included in many different liniments and arthritis rubs including Ben-Gay ointment, Icy Hot cream, and Aspercreme cream. These products are called counterirritants because they create a sensation of heat when applied to the skin, sometimes confusing pain impulses derived from deeper tissues. It may also increase blood flow to the area where it is applied, removing toxins that produce pain. The substance should never be taken orally. It is safe when used appropriately.

Cloves (Syzygium aromaticum)

Cloves are the dried, dark brown unexpanded flower buds of an evergreen tree found in the tropics. Used commonly as a spice, cloves also contain oil that can be extracted through steam distillation from the buds, stems, and leaves. The oil is reported to have pain-relieving properties. A tea can be made using the oil that may also relieve nausea, as well as treat upset stomach, gas, sore throat, and dental pain. For thousands of years, Chinese healers used cloves to treat a variety of health conditions ranging from diarrhea to hernias. A few drops of clove oil are used to make the tea. Mouthwashes are made using concentrations of oil from 1 to 5 percent. The undiluted oil can be applied directly to painful teeth or mouth sores. Safety is not proven and potency of commercial preparations may vary widely.

Cinnamon (Cinnamomum zeylanicum *Blume*)

Cinnamon comes from the dried bark of the *Cinnamomum zeylanicum* tree found growing in the West Indies and Asia. Oils are extracted from the leaves, bark, stems, and roots. Ancient Egyptians and Chinese healers used cinnamon to treat upset stomach, abdominal pain, painful menstruation, and arthritis. Today it is used for these problems, as well as to relieve nausea and other digestive complaints. Cinnamon can be bought in health food stores as a capsule, oil, powder, tea bag, or tincture. A solution is made using one teaspoon per cup of water ingested two or three times per day with meals. Cinnamon can also be taken as a capsule of dried bark at a dose of 2 grams once or twice daily. Safety is not proven and potency of commercial preparations may vary widely.

Cod-Liver Oil

This concentrated oil is obtained from the codfish and contains high amounts of vitamins A and D but is low in saturated fatty acids. Cod-liver oil is a good source of omega-3 fatty acids (OFA). OFAs may lower cholesterol, reduce inflammation from arthritis, and may act as a blood thinner. Cod-liver oil is taken at an average dose of 1 to 2 tablespoons daily. Capsules are also available. Safety is not proven and potency of commercial preparations may vary widely.

Devil's Claw (Harpagophytum procumbens)

Devil's claw grows wild in the deserts and steppes of southern Africa. It gets its name from its fruit, the tips of which have small barbs or claws. The secondary roots (sometimes called storage tubers) are used to treat arthritis and problems with digestion. Devil's claw supposedly helps to promote flexibility in painful arthritic joints. It is available in capsules, liquid extract, and chopped or powdered root. The recommended dose is 4.5 grams per day, which is taken as a drink made from 1 teaspoon powdered or chopped root mixed in two cups of water. Safety is not proven and potency of commercial preparations may vary widely.

Ivy (Hedera helix)

This well-known climbing plant can be found anywhere in the United States, especially in northern climates. Its leaves are used either fresh or crushed into a watery solution, or can be made into a poultice. Incisions made in the bark of the ivy plant will yield a substance known as ivy gum; both this and the black berries of the plant have been used to treat various ailments. Herbalists once recommended ivy for arthritis and rheumatism. A poultice made of ivy leaves or gum may be applied externally to treat burns or skin diseases. The gum has also been reported to relieve toothache by applying it directly to the tooth. A solution can be made for internal use by pouring boiling water over about 0.5 grams of fresh or dried ivy leaves, letting it sit for ten minutes, and straining off the leaves to make a drink that is ingested from one to three times a day. Safety is not proven and potency of commercial preparations may vary widely.

Mustard (Brassica)

This plant yields seeds that, after ripening and drying, are supposed to be effective for pain relief. Mustard oil can also be made from the seeds. The seeds and the oil have been used externally for the treatment of joint pain, joint inflammation, and pain in the lower back or lumbar region. Mustard is sold as a liniment, oil, ointment, paste, plaster, or poultice. Two handfuls of ground mustard seed are mixed with lukewarm water to make a paste that is spread on a cloth, placed on the painful joint, and removed after a strong burning sensation is felt. Mustard oil may also be applied to the skin over a painful joint in concentrations of 0.5 to 5 percent at a frequency of three to four times daily. Safety is not proven and potency of commercial preparations may vary widely.

Capsaicin

The active ingredient in hot peppers that makes them hot, capsaicin has been used for thousands of years in Mexico for many purposes in religious and healing ceremonies. When applied to the skin, it causes a warm or burning sensation, which led to its use in liniments and arthritis rubs, such as Heet. Although the effects of capsaicin on pain had long been thought to result from its counterirritant properties, it is now known that capsaicin depletes nerve endings of substance P, one of the neurochemicals thought to transmit pain sensations to the brain. Many preparations exist including Capzasin-P, Dolorac, Zostrix, and Zostrix-HP, which are over-the-counter remedies for arthritis, muscle aches, postherpetic neuralgia, and peripheral neuropathies.

Epsom Salt

First discovered in the mineral-rich waters of Epsom, England, Epsom salt is the popular term for the chemical magnesium sulfate. When dissolved in warm water, it tends to create a gentle drawing action that can reduce the swelling, muscle ache, and pain resulting from bruised or irritated tissues, as well as draw out toxins. Often used as a foot soak, it can also be used in full-body baths.

Gin-Soaked Raisins

This treatment has for many years been suggested as a home remedy for the treatment of arthritis pain. One box of golden light raisins is layered at the bottom of a 10-inch by 16-inch pan. A pint of gin is poured over the raisins to completely cover them. The raisins must be allowed to sit uncovered immersed in gin for approximately seven days until the gin completely evaporates. Recommended dose is to eat nine raisins per day for pain relief. If there is no relief after one or two months, then future benefits are unlikely. There may be scientific reasons for the benefits of this treatment. Raisins contain a certain amount of pain-relieving salicylate (the active ingredient in aspirin), which the gin may help to concentrate. No studies have examined the effectiveness of this method, although there are plenty of testimonies from individuals that it works (for humans and animals!).[6]

St. John's Wort

Studies done in Europe over the past several decades have produced a lot of information about St. John's wort. Those studies show this herbal supplement to be a promising drug for treating depression, including depression associated with chronic pain. There is need for caution, however, for patients taking medications such as tetracycline, cyclosporin, protease inhibitors, digoxin, warfarin, oral birth control pills, and drugs to treat asthma. There is evidence that St. John's wort may cause certain enzymes in the liver to process these medications faster than usual, resulting in lower levels in the body. There is also concern with photosensitivity, in that severe sunburns may occur if St. John's wort is taken before prolonged exposure to the sun.

Finally, many of the preparations of St. John's wort available over the counter do not have sufficient amounts of the active ingredient (hypericin or hyperforin) to have an effect. A recent study conducted by ConsumerLab.com, an independent evaluator of dietary supplements and nutrition products, examined twenty-one brands of St. John's wort available over the counter.[7] Five of these products had insufficient levels of the active ingredient necessary to have therapeutic effects. Furthermore, five of the brands also exceeded the safe limit for cadmium, a known cancer-producing element and potential toxin. They recommended that labels be examined carefully to identify the amount of hypericin or hyperforin the product contains.

A number of recent studies have examined the effectiveness of St. John's wort in treating depression. The first large U.S. clinical trial involving 200 patients with moderate to severe depression released its results in 2001. No significant difference in response rates was found between those receiving St. John's wort and those receiving placebo (27 percent got better with the drug and 19 percent with placebo).[8] In the largest trial to date, a multisite NIH study, 340 adult outpatients with major depression were randomly assigned to receive St. John's wort, placebo, or sertraline (Zoloft) for eight weeks. The daily dose of St. John's wort ranged from 900 to 1,500 mg and that of sertraline from 50 to 100 mg. On both primary outcome measures, St. John's wort failed to perform better than placebo (32 percent response rate for placebo versus 24 percent response rate for St. John's wort). The authors concluded that St. John's wort was not effective for moderately severe depression.[9] Therefore, if people are suffering symptoms of depression, they should not self-medicate, but should instead consult a physician. No studies have yet examined the effects of St. John's wort on chronic pain in the absence of depression.

Omega-3 Fatty Acids

For persons with arthritis pain, reduction of inflammation may be achieved by increasing intake of omega-3 fatty acids (eicosapentaenoic acid [EPA], decosahexanoic acid [DHA], and alpha-linoleic acid [ALA]),[10] which may also improve mood if depression is a problem. This can be done by consuming fish often (salmon, trout, or tuna) or flaxseeds (ground up and made into bread or pancakes, sprinkled on food, or used as flaxseed butter). Use of flaxseed oil and canola oil for cooking will also increase intake of omega-3 fatty acids. A number of tasty recipes for dishes high in omega-3 fatty acids can be prepared.[11] Unfortunately, very large amounts of fish and flaxseeds must be consumed to achieve the levels necessary for therapeutic effects (between six and thirty-two cans of tuna per day, for example).

Alternatively, fish oil supplements (capsules) containing EPA and DHA can be taken at doses of 2 to 5 g daily, although further benefit may be seen at doses as high as 10 g/day (note that the traditional diet of Greenland Eskimos includes up to 14 g/day). Fish oil preparations vary from 30 percent to 90 percent in their omega-3 fatty acid content (a 1 g capsule of Fish Body oils by GNC contains 30 percent or 300 mg, whereas 500 mg capsules of Omega-Brite by Omega Natural Science in Waltham, Massachusetts, contain 90 percent or 450 mg). With the GNC product, four capsules twice daily are necessary to achieve a minimum dose of 2 g per day and up to eight to ten capsules twice daily to reach doses of 5-6 g per day. Alternatively, two tablespoons (30 cc's) of flaxseed oil per day provide 10 grams of ALA (alha-linolenic acid).

Side effects of excessive omega-3 fatty acid intake, although rare and related to dose, may include nausea and occasional diarrhea, symptoms of excessive vitamin A intake (hair loss, liver problems, etc.), and impaired platelet function (causing increased bleeding). If taking flaxseeds or flaxmeal, do not take more than 2-3 tablespoons per day because seed husks contain toxic ingredients that can build up in the system. People who are taking blood thinners such as aspirin or warfarin (Coumadin) need to check with their doctors before taking omega-3 fatty acid supplements.

GLUCOSAMINE AND CHONDROITIN SULFATE

Glucosamine sulfate, used either alone or in combination with chondroitin sulfate, is reported to significantly reduce the pain of arthritis. A recent review of the research examining the effectiveness of glucosamine and chondroitin sulfate in osteoarthritis was published in the *Journal of the American Medical Association (JAMA).*[12] In this review, fifteen double-blind, randomized, placebo-controlled studies that lasted four weeks or more were analyzed (nearly all the studies were conducted between 1966 and 1999). The average benefit (expressed in terms of "effect size") was a significant 0.44 (95 percent confidence interval [CI], 0.24-0.64) for glucosamine and 0.78 (95 percent CI, 0.60-0.95) for chondroitin. Benefits were consistent for pain and ability to function, although effects weakened when only high-quality or large studies were considered.

The investigators concluded that glucosamine and chondroitin sulfate for use in osteoarthritis produced moderate to large effects, but that the quality of the studies was poor and these effects were likely exaggerated. They did admit, however, that some degree of effective pain relief and increased function was likely with the use of these products. Bear in mind that most studies were relatively short (a few months at most) and that the long-term benefits and toxic side effects of glucosamine and chondroitin have not been determined. Also, the purity and content of glucosamine and chondroitin in different preparations is not standardized and may differ considerably since these products are not regulated by the FDA. Toxic side effects may also vary by preparation.

The most impressive study performed to date examined 212 patients with osteoarthritis of the knee who were randomly assigned in a double-blind fashion to receive either 1,500 mg glucosamine sulfate once a day or a placebo for three years. At the start of the study, the two groups of 106 patients were similar in terms of age, sex, and severity of disease. Subjects receiving the placebo experienced significant joint space deterioration during follow-up, whereas no joint space deterioration occurred in the glucosamine sulfate group. The investigators concluded that placebo-treated patients experienced a slight worsening in symptoms at the end of the study, compared to an improvement in those who had received glucosamine sulfate.[13]

The National Institutes of Health is now sponsoring one of the largest studies ever to evaluate glucosamine and chondroitin for the treatment of osteoarthritis.[14] This study is a sixteen-week, double-blind randomized clinical trial that includes four treatment arms, in which patients will receive either a placebo (sugar pill), 500 mg glucosamine sulfate three times per day, 400 mg chondroitin sulfate three times per day, or a combination of glucosamine and chondroitin. Results of this study are not yet published.

Those considering taking glucosamine supplements should be aware that the dose used in clinical trials is typically 500 mg three times daily. For chondroitin sulfate, the typical dose is 400 mg three times daily. Other substances claimed to have natural anti-inflammatory effects include Catherine's Choice, Bromelain in pineapple stalk, Arthro-7

(Gero Vita), methyl sulfonyl methane (MSM), and cetyl myristoleate (CMO). Few reliable studies have been performed on these preparations, making it difficult to recommend them.

ALTERNATIVE MEDICAL PROCEDURES

According to an American Geriatrics Society consensus panel,[15] alternative therapies are widely used for the treatment of pain in the United States, although physicians are frequently not informed by patients of their use. As noted earlier, these treatments can be expensive and may deplete economic resources that could be used for proven treatments. Although such treatments offer hope, their usual lack of effectiveness often results in disillusionment and emotional upset. Nevertheless, when traditional therapies are not effective, patients seek relief outside the traditional health care system. Many persons with chronic pain report at least temporary relief using one or more of the following treatments.

Acupuncture

Originating in China during the Xia Dynasty (2140-1711 B.C.), acupuncture is based on the concept that a continuous flow of chi ("life energy") exists which is closely connected with human health. Acupuncture seeks to improve health by placing needles at specific points on the skin to release and enhance the flow of chi. In the United States, the procedure gained notoriety when public figure and well-known columnist James Reston in 1971 underwent an emergency appendectomy in Beijing and afterward described the effectiveness of acupuncture in relieving his pain. Today, Americans make 12 million visits to acupuncturists each year. Acupuncture is said to be particularly effective in relieving the pain associated with fibromyalgia. Patients do not usually experience pain during acupuncture. Treatments typically last from five to thirty minutes and anywhere from one to twenty needles are used. Most patients require at least three treatments. Side effects during treatment, although rare, include fainting, bruising, pain, infection, and damage to underlying tissues.

Acupuncture is one of the oldest forms of treatment based on ancient Chinese religious and philosophical tradition. It is heavily emphasized in traditional Chinese medicine. The effectiveness of acupuncture is based on restoring the balance between yin and yang forces within the body. According to ancient Chinese philosophy, lifeforce energy (chi) circulates throughout the body along meridians that have yin or yang characteristics. There are 361 acupuncture points along these meridians that when activated are believed to correct the imbalance of yin and yang responsible for disease (and pain). Many different forms of acupuncture have evolved in Western culture, including Japanese meridian therapy, French energetic acupuncture, Korean acupuncture, Lemington acupuncture, ear acupuncture, scalp acupuncture, and hand and foot acupuncture.

Those who practice acupuncture today may insert needles in additional points not located along traditional meridians, including trigger points where tenderness is felt. Various forms of stimulation include needles as well as electrical acupuncture (where needles are stimulated with electricity), injection acupuncture (where herbs are injected), and moxibustion acupuncture (where *Artemis vulgaris,* a special herb, is burned at the end of the needle).

The exact physiological mechanism by which acupuncture has its supposed effects is not well known (other than promoting the flow of chi through the body). Some research suggests that a biological mechanism does exist for pain relief during acupuncture. According to the gate-control theory of pain, activation of small nerve fibers in the skin sends impulses to the spinal cord, midbrain, pituitary, and hypothalamus, which inhibits the transmission of pain. It has also been claimed that acupuncture may stimulate production of neurotransmitters such as serotonin, acetylcholine, and other substances such as endorphins (opiatelike substances made by the body that relieve pain). Besides distracting the nervous system from areas of underlying pain or stimulating the production of endorphins, acupuncture may work by inducing subtle magnetic field changes or altering subtle body energies; none of these explanations, however, is widely accepted by scientists since research supporting these claims is sparse.[16]

Acupuncture is reported to provide short-term benefits for 50 to 70 percent of people with chronic pain, and some long-term effects may also be experienced in selected cases. Is this a placebo effect? Placebo pills achieve pain relief in 30 to 35 percent of cases and sham ("pretend") acupuncture with instruments and rituals is effective in about 50 percent of subjects. Whether acupuncture takes care of an underlying problem or has only a psychological benefit, however, is less important than the fact that it may help some people feel better. An expert consensus panel convened by the National Institutes of Health in 1997 concluded that evidence exists for acupuncture's effectiveness in relieving pain after dental surgery, and that it may be useful for osteoarthritis, low back pain, headache (both tension and migraine), menstrual cramps, carpal tunnel syndrome, fibromyalgia, and other conditions that cause chronic pain. The research supporting that conclusion, though, is less than solid.

Ter Riet and colleagues conducted a literature search that identified fifty-one controlled clinical studies on the effectiveness of acupuncture in treating chronic pain. These investigators found that the quality of even some of the better studies was poor, and the results from those studies were highly contradictory. The authors concluded, "the efficacy of acupuncture in the treatment of chronic pain remains doubtful" (p. 1191).[17] More recently, Van Tulder and colleagues conducted a systematic review of the literature on the usefulness of acupuncture in the treatment of low back pain.[18] These investigators identified and reviewed eleven randomized controlled trials. Based on this review they concluded there was "no evidence showing acupuncture to be more effective than no treatment" (p. 1113) and did not recommend acupuncture be used as a regular treatment for patients with low back pain.

Energy Medicine

A variety of contraptions and procedures exist that are best categorized under what has been called *energy medicine*. Most of these are extremely controversial and unproven. Some techniques are electrified versions of therapies such as acupuncture. Others are derived from electrical treatments originating in the nineteenth century. None of these forms of energy therapy have been tested or verified by scientific research, although several studies are ongoing. Examples include electroacupuncture, auricular acupuncture (acupuncture applied to the ear), microcurrent electrical therapy, and a number of devices such as the electro-acuscope, light beam generator, cymatic devices, sound probe, and diapulse. In 1975, A. Franz Morell, working in conjunction with a bioelectronic engineer, Erich Rasche, introduced the MORA-Therapy Unit" (MOrell + RAsche = MORA). The MORA unit supposedly delivers electromagnetic energy to various acupuncture points, thereby helping to relieve headaches and muscular aches and pains. The electro-acuscope and microcurrent electrical therapy supposedly relieve pain of muscle spasms, headaches, bursitis, and arthritis by running electric current through damaged tissues. Cymatic devices use sound and radio waves tuned to the "frequency" of various body organs or tissues to restore health. For example, a diapulse machine employs radio waves to reduce swelling and inflammation. There is little if any published research to substantiate the claims made for any of these devices.

Alexander Technique

The Alexander technique (AT), which attempts to bring the body's muscles into natural harmony, has been used in the treatment of neurological and musculoskeletal disorders of the neck, back, and hip; traumatic and repetitive strain injuries; chronic arthritis; and headache. Persons with sciatica, osteoporosis, osteoarthritis, rheumatoid arthritis, and neck or low back pain may find the AT useful in improving strength and mobility. It may also be used in fibromyalgia to manage pain. Sessions are usually conducted one on one with a therapist, although AT can be conducted in groups as well. The subject is asked to perform everyday actions, such as walking, bending, standing, or sitting, while the therapist encourages the person to shed ingrained unhealthy muscular reactions and replace them with healthy natural reflexes. The therapist may lead the person through various movements, touching the neck, back, or shoulder to trigger the proper reflexes. AT can be directed at improving certain movements or actions, such as working at a computer, holding a telephone, or driving a car. Although AT is not a passive experience such as a massage, sessions are not physically strenuous and no mechanical devices are used. No scientific studies have yet examined the efficacy of this technique, so benefits of AT are unsubstantiated.

Aston-Patterning

Aston-Patterning (AP) is a program of bodywork and movement training aimed at relieving muscle tension, pain, and speeding recovery from injury. AP can be used for back and neck pain, headache, and repetitive stress injuries. AP sessions are conducted with a trained therapist and include massage, movement training, fitness exercises, and advice on changes in the home and work environments. As part of the evaluation process, actions such as sitting, standing, and walking are examined, and efforts are made to correct movements that are considered abnormal. AP focuses on flexion and extension exercises to improve posture and other movements. The massage element of the treatment involves a special "spiraling" technique that relaxes tense muscles and loosens stiff joints. Repetitive exercises are used to reinforce the results of massage and to correct posture and gait so healthy movements become natural. Improved muscle tone, joint resiliency, and lightness of movement are primary goals. Psychological counseling is used to reinforce healthy movement and posture. Advice is given on how to make changes in the environment to maintain healthy posture by changing the height of a chair and using cushions, knee supports, and even side body supports to keep the spine and other areas of the body in proper alignment. AP has not been studied scientifically, and no objective evidence of its effectiveness exists.

Feldenkrais Method

The Feldenkrais method is considered by its practitioners to be useful for a variety of chronic pains, including headache, joint disorders, and neck, shoulder, and back pain. It may also help those with chronic neuromuscular disorders, such as multiple sclerosis or cerebral palsy, and may benefit those who have suffered from a stroke. The technique may help to improve balance, coordination, and mobility. The method has two components. One is called functional integration and consists of hands-on sessions by a practitioner who uses touch to help improve physical movement patterns. While the person is sitting, standing, or reclining, the practitioner will manipulate his or her muscles and joints, as done by others who perform similar types of bodywork. Feldenkrais manipulations, however, are all carried out within the usual range of motion and without pain or the forceful bending of joints.

The second component of this method is training to increase the person's awareness of other movements by focusing on everyday movements such as sitting and standing. The functional integration sessions usually last about forty-five minutes, whereas the awareness sessions last forty-five to sixty minutes; a complete treatment course involves four to six weekly sessions. It has not yet been scientifically studied, so this treatment method has not been proven effective.

Hellerwork

Another type of bodywork, Hellerwork, involves a combination of deep tissue massage and retraining in body movement. It may help conditions associated with muscle tension and stress—especially pain in the back, neck, or shoulders. More specifically, Hellerwork therapy consists of a series of sessions during which a practitioner helps the individual get in touch with his or her emotions and related body parts. The first session, lasting about ninety minutes, involves working on the upper body to release tensions that interfere with normal breathing. Prior to doing anything physical with the patient, the practitioner talks with him or her to identify emotional attitudes that may be interfering with normal body movements. Next, the practitioner uses physical manipulation of the muscles to help release built-up tensions. The goal of treatment is to help the person achieve a better understanding of the relationship between the mind and body, which practitioners claim is usually accomplished in ten or eleven sessions.

Hydrotherapy

Throughout most of recorded history water has been used in the treatment of a wide variety of ailments, particularly musculoskeletal injuries, back pain, arthritis, menstrual cramps, diabetes, and other diseases associated with impaired circulation. For example, the application of hot or cold water compresses to manage pain and tissue swelling is common today. Physical therapy for those with weak or painful joints is often performed in heated pools. Even psychiatric patients were for many years treated with hydrotherapy as a way of calming excitement or irritability. Less widely accepted forms of hydrotherapy performed by alternative medicine practitioners today involve techniques such as constitutional hydrotherapy and hot fomentation, which are designed to rid the body of its toxins. None of these methods has been subject to scientific testing for effectiveness.

Constitutional hydrotherapy involves the systematic application of hot and cold wet towels to the body, together with the administration of mild electrical stimulation to large muscle groups. The patient rests on an examination table on his or her back. The therapist covers the patient's upper body with two hot, moist towels at a temperature of about 120°F. After about five minutes, a new set of hot towels is placed over the original ones. The towels are then flipped over so that the fresh, hotter ones are against the body. Next, cold towels are placed over the hot towels and then flipped so that the cold towels lie against the body. The cold towels remain in place on the chest for ten minutes. During the time the cold wet towels are in place, the practitioner places an electrical pad on either side of the person's spine just below the shoulders to deliver a mild, nonpainful electrical current to the back muscles for about ten minutes. After that, the therapist removes the cold towels and repositions the pads so one is located at the center of the lower back area and the other on the abdomen in the solar plexus region, applying the electrical current for another ten minutes. The process described is then repeated with the person lying on his or her stomach. The treatment ends with the practitioner rubbing down the patient's body with a dry towel. The whole process lasts about an hour and is usually repeated on a schedule of two to three times per week for up to fifteen sessions.

Hot fomentation is similar to constitutional hydrotherapy except it does not include the electrical muscle stimulation. In this procedure, hot moist towels are again applied to the body (often to the part or parts causing pain), sometimes with special herbs included in the water in which towels are soaked. Besides lying down on an examining table, the patient may also place his or her feet in hot water while the hot towels are in place. The final part of the treatment involves a rubdown with a cold towel after the hot towels are removed.

Hypnotherapy

A now accepted form of behavioral therapy (see Chapter 10), hypnosis has been used as a treatment for pain since around 1850 (and was likely used long before that). This procedure is based upon suggestions and exercises given during a state of deep, conscious relaxation. Hypnosis can improve relaxation, sleep, energy level, and decrease pain. During a typical visit, the patient first discusses his or her problems and pain with the therapist to build trust and rapport. Deep-breathing exercises are initiated, and the patient is guided into relaxation of each body part. In the deep relaxed state that results, the subconscious mind is open to receiving beneficial suggestions that have been agreed upon between patient and therapist before the session. There may be suggestions to change behaviors, thoughts, and feelings. Because patients are aware throughout the session, they may learn to do this independently on their own. Hypnosis typically takes place in a quiet setting with muted lights, a comfortable chair, and no interruptions. The session will usually last about twenty to sixty minutes. The number of sessions is correlated with degree of improvement. Studies have shown that hypnosis is more effective than placebo and that those who can relax more easily achieve the best results. This technique is most effective for persons with fibromyalgia (myofacial pain syndrome) or headache.

Therapeutic Touch

Therapeutic touch (TT) is an Eastern spiritual technique rooted in mysticism involving the "laying on" of hands to induce an energy transfer or to activate the inner healer. It is widely used in the practice of holistic nursing. This technique is believed to restore balance in the human energy field, promote relaxation, and reduce pain.[19] TT involves moving both hands (called "hand passes") approximately two to six inches above the person's body from head to feet; this method is used for both diagnosing and rectifying imbalances in the patient's energy field. Research on therapeutic touch has been sorely lacking, and most of the studies done are reported in the *Journal of Holistic Nursing*. Benefits are often assessed by comparing before and after measures of depression, anxiety, and pain; control groups and statistical methodology in such studies are seldom adequate. Even a reviewer favorable to the technique concluded that no congruence was found among investigators on how to measure the effects of TT, that most of the research designs had not been replicated, and that research on the usefulness of therapeutic touch was inconclusive.[20]

An interesting test of TT did, however, make it into a prominent medical journal (JAMA). Rosa and colleagues comprehensively reviewed the literature and reported the results of a clinical trial to assess the effectiveness of therapeutic touch.[21] These investigators examined whether TT practitioners could actually perceive a "human energy field" with their hands. Their sample consisted of twenty-one practitioners with TT experience ranging from one to twenty-seven years. The practitioners were tested under blinded conditions to determine whether they could correctly identify which of their hands was closest to one of the investigator's hands. Fourteen of the practitioners were tested ten times each, and seven practitioners were tested twenty times each. Practitioners were asked to indicate whether the investigator's unseen hand hovered above their right hand or their left hand. A score of 50 percent would be expected on the basis of chance alone. The results indicated that practitioners identified the correct hand only 44 percent of the time, which is actually less often than would be expected by chance. Length of practitioner experience was not correlated with practitioners' score. Investigators found that practitioners of TT could not reliably detect a human energy field, thus failing to substantiate TT's most fundamental claim. They concluded that the claims of TT were groundless and did not justify further professional use of this technique.

Massage Therapy

Many different types of massage exist, including specialized treatments ranging from reflexology to shiatsu (not covered here). Most massage practitioners, however, apply five basic strokes: effleurage, petrissage, friction, percussion, and vibration and jostling. Effleurage is the use of the palm, fingers, or knuckles to produce slow, rhythmic strokes usually directed from the extremities toward the center of the body. Petrissage involves the grasping and releasing of muscle tissue in pressing and rolling movements. Friction is the application of pressure or circular movements across muscle groups without moving across the skin (usually done for muscles around joints). Percussion involves beating with the side of the hand, cupping the fingers and striking with the heel of the hand, or clapping with a flat hand across the large muscle groups of the back. Finally, vibration involves rapid movements of the therapist's hands or mechanical vibrators to shake the muscles; jostling is similar and involves a rapid back-and-forth shaking of the muscles. These five strokes help to relax muscles and increase blood flow, carrying away toxins that produce pain. Other forms involve neuromuscular massage in which the therapist applies finger pressure to painful trigger points over muscles. Deep tissue massage involves firm, deep strokes with the fingers over tense muscles, especially across the neck or shoulder.

Rolfing

Rolfing consists of deep, sometimes painful muscle massage. It has been used as therapy for chronic back pain, whiplash, and spinal problems. Rolfing seeks to loosen and relax the membranes that surround the muscles (fascia) which may thicken and knot up with time and tension. To break out the knots in the fascia, practitioners of Rolfing apply slow, sliding pressure to the muscles with their knuckles, thumbs, fingers, and sometimes even elbows and knees. Rolfing treatments often induce pain in the short run, yet promising relief over the long term because the body is brought back into more proper alignment. Treatments are performed with the patient sitting or lying, and manipulations may be synchronized with the patient's breathing. The therapist focuses on a particular set of muscles during each 60 to 90 minute session, starting first with muscles near the surface and then moving on to deeper muscles.

Magnet Therapy

Some scientific evidence suggests that certain pain conditions may benefit from magnet therapy. Brown presented data from a small study of eight patients with chronic pelvic pain at the annual meeting of the American College of Obstetrics and Gynecology in May 2000.[22] Investigators placed magnets on two trigger points on the abdomen that elicited pain when pressure was applied. Sixty percent of women treated with magnets experienced a reduction in pain compared to 33 percent of women given "sham" or inactive magnets. Whether this difference was statistically significant was not mentioned. It is not known why the application of magnets would reduce pain; however, magnets may somehow increase blood flow or interfere with nerves conducting painful stimuli.

These same investigators are now repeating the study with a larger group of thirty women to determine whether they can replicate their results. Other studies, however, have not found magnet therapy to be effective. According to a study published in JAMA, magnet therapy produced no greater results than did sham treatment in twenty people with chronic back pain.[23] Subjects were randomly assigned to treatment with either a real magnet or a sham magnet that had been demagnetized. The study was double-blinded, meaning that neither the patients nor the investigators knew who received the real magnets. Subjects wore either the real or the sham magnet over the area of pain for six hours a day on Monday, Wednesday, and Friday. The magnets were then taken off for one week and the treatment and sham groups switched appliances, which were then worn for another three days in the same manner.

Although neither the real nor the sham magnets produced any significant pain relief, there were no side effects to the treatment either. Study investigators indicated that perhaps stronger magnets were needed for the treatment of back pain. For those who were currently receiving benefit from magnet therapy, investigators encouraged continued use.

Chiropractic

Chiropractic is a form of spinal manipulation that chiropractors use most commonly to treat acute lower back pain. Chiropractic manipulations may also be helpful in some cases of chronic pain related to back, neck, or peripheral joint problems, and may be used as a treatment for headaches. There is evidence that spinal manipulation can help many people. Even the U.S. government's Agency for Health Care Policy and Research (AHCPR) promoted the technique's use in its *Guidelines on Acute Low Back Problems in Adults,** indicating that spinal manipulation is the preferred method of treatment for relief of *acute* back pain substantiated in part by a recent clinical trial published in the *New England Journal of Medicine*.[24] At least one major clinical trial, however, did not find the technique useful for headache.[25] Although no scientific studies confirm its use for any-

---

*See Web site: <http://www.amerchiro.org/media/faqs.shtml> to obtain a copy of these guidelines.

thing but low back pain, studies are now being conducted under the sponsorship of the NIH's Office of Alternative Medicine to see whether other conditions might be treated using this method.

SUMMARY AND CONCLUSIONS

Many alternative and complementary treatments exist for chronic pain, and it is difficult to know which treatment is worth pursuing, if any. My general recommendation is that it usually doesn't hurt to try one of these alternative treatments, particularly if it isn't too expensive. If clear benefits are not evident after two or three months of use, or if the initial benefit is not sustained over time, then the treatment should be stopped. In general, the placebo effect usually works for about two or three months whether the treatment is effective or not. After that, the effectiveness of a placebo begins to diminish.

I've tried a number of alternative treatments for my arthritis pain. These include magnets, fish oil pills with omega-3 fatty acids, glucosamine, gin-soaked raisins, and a gelatin dietary supplement. I applied the magnets to my wrists and also inserted magnetized pads into my shoes. The magnets appeared to work for a time, but then lost their effectiveness, so I stopped them without noticeable worsening. The only treatments I continue now are the fish oil pills (4 g/day), because it is also likely to benefit my cardiovascular system and is not very expensive, and 1,000 mg glucosamine twice daily.

Chapter 12

Surgical and Other Procedures

This chapter examines surgical treatments and other procedures used to alleviate chronic pain. It focuses primarily on conditions not due to cancer or other terminal illness. Surgery can be very useful for acute conditions that cause pain, such as gallbladder disease, kidney stones, protrusion of a herniated disc, or problems due to diseases of the blood vessels. The same is true for terminal conditions in which pain is severe and an operation may help bring relief. For chronic nonmalignant pain, however, surgery seldom brings lasting relief without complications. Pain often recurs in the long run, and the severing of nerve pathways may lead to weakness or loss of urinary or bowel control. This does not, however, mean that surgery is never helpful for persons with chronic pain, but only that the decision to have surgery should be made after careful consideration and weighing of benefits and risks.

Although surgical procedures for the relief of chronic pain are often a treatment of last resort, there are times when an appropriate surgical procedure can produce lasting relief while at the same time avoiding many of the side effects and complications associated with long-term medication use. For example, treatment of the excruciating facial pain from trigeminal neuralgia that results from a small blood vessel pressing up against a nerve located close to the brain involves surgical removal of the blood vessel or placement of a small cushion between the nerve and the vessel, which can bring lasting pain relief. Likewise, for a person with a deteriorated hip or knee joint from degenerative arthritis, replacement of the diseased knee or hip with an artificial joint can bring great relief and return of function. Unfortunately, surgery is often not helpful for people who have chronic low back pain, bone or joint pain, muscle pain, or headache. As a result, many of the traditional neurosurgical procedures for the management of chronic pain are used sparingly these days. With this note of caution, the various types of neurosurgical and orthopedic procedures that are useful in the treatment of chronic pain are examined next.

NEUROSURGERY

Neurosurgery involves the cutting or destruction (ablation) of peripheral nerves, nerve pathways in the spinal cord, or pain-sensing areas of the brain to relieve severe, unrelenting pain that cannot be made tolerable by drugs or other less drastic measures.[1]

Peripheral Nerve Block

In certain places on the body, nerves are easily accessible to injection with a local anesthetic. This procedure is based on the notion that temporarily blocking nerve function can bring relief from pain or muscle spasm. Nerve endings deeply imbedded in skin, muscles, bone, or internal organs transmit pain impulses along their axons to the spinal cord or brainstem, and then to the brain. If the function of these nerves can be interrupted somewhere along their pathways, this will help prevent the pain signals from reaching the brain. This interruption of nerve function is temporary and accomplished by numbing or blocking the nerve through the injection of a local anesthetic. Peripheral nerve blocks can also be used diagnostically to identify from where pain is originating. For example, if pain is caused by a problem in the spinal cord or brain, then blocking a peripheral nerve will cause the area to feel numb, but will not relieve the pain.

Peripheral nerve blocks must be done with considerable care. If the physician injects the numbing medicine (lidocaine) directly into the nerve, this will cause extreme pain during the injection and may even lead to the formation of a small nerve tumor within the nerve itself (called a neuroma), which itself can lead to chronic pain.

Nerve blocks have long been discouraged in patients with no identifiable organic abnormality (medical or biological cause for the pain) and in those whose disability and discomfort appear worse than would be expected based on the known physical damage or injury.[2] Nerve blocks should also never be administered as an isolated procedure for patients with chronic pain, but rather as part of a broader pain management program. This is particularly true for patients in whom nerve-block procedures and pain clinic management have not been effective in the past.

Nerve Destruction

Irreversible neurolytic techniques involve the permanent cutting, chemical destruction, or high frequency radio wave or laser-induced ablation of nerve bodies or pathways. The sophistication of neuro-ablation has increased with the use of computers that can now pinpoint the location of nerves responsible for pain. These procedures are largely reserved today for persons who are terminally ill, given the permanent loss of function that often results. The use of these procedures for chronic benign pain remains highly controversial. The introduction of radiofrequency techniques, however, has broadened the usefulness of neuroablation in the treatment of chronic pain. This method allows for a localized area of nerve destruction without risk of damaging surrounding tissues, as previously occurred with phenol or alcohol injections. Radiofrequency neurolytic techniques are now being considered for the treatment of low back pain and other sources of chronic pain.

Sympathectomy

This procedure involves the permanent cutting or chemical destruction of sympathetic nerve fibers responsible for certain kinds of pain syndromes such as causalgia (burning pain and hypersensitivity due to damage to sympathetic nerves from injury or disease) and reflex sympathetic dystrophy (continuous pain in all or a portion of an extremity that does not involve a major nerve, often resulting in a painful cold extremity with severe muscle wasting). Sympathetic nerve fibers may also be responsible for pain from postherpetic neuralgia (chronic pain following infection with the herpes zoster virus) and certain perineal pain syndromes (pain in the area of the genitals and anus). If temporary blocking of sympathetic nerve fibers reduces the pain, then a neurolytic procedure may be performed to destroy the part of the sympathetic nervous system responsible for the pain.

Destruction of Spinal Roots

Spinal roots consist of bundles of nerves entering into and going out of the spinal cord. These nerve roots may be pressed on by a protruding vertebral disc, bony spur, or cancerous tumor resulting in chronic pain. Even after spinal operations that remove the disc or bony spur, pain from the irritated spinal root may continue. Chemical ablation of the spinal root may help relieve pain, although this also destroys the function of the body part innervated by the nerves involved. In terminal cases, this loss of function may be worth the pain relief obtained.

Cordotomy

In extreme cases, almost always restricted to persons with end-stage cancer suffering severe unrelenting pain, an operation may be done to sever a portion of the spinal cord in order to interrupt the nerve pathways that transmit pain to the brain. During cordotomy, a specific nerve pathway (the anterolateral spinothalamic tract) is cut to produce loss of pain and temperature sensations on the opposite side of the body. Patients with severe one-sided pain arising from tumors in the chest wall, abdomen, or lower extremity are most likely to benefit. Recent advances in technique now allow this procedure to be done percutaneously through a small incision in the skin without requiring major back surgery. Open cordotomy (major back surgery) is usually reserved for patients who are unable to lie on their stomachs or who are not cooperative enough to undergo the percutaneous procedure.

Pain relief has been achieved in more than 90 percent of patients during the period immediately following the procedure, although after twelve months 50 percent experience recurrent pain. Neurologic complications of the procedure may include paralysis, dizziness, difficulty walking, and loss of bladder control. In about 5 percent of patients these complications are protracted and disabling. The most serious complication from the procedure is paralysis of the nerves that control breathing, particularly in patients who undergo high bilateral cordotomy (where both the left and right anterolateral spinothalamic tracts are severed).

Cordectomy is a more aggressive procedure that involves the removal of the lower end of the spinal cord in cases of severe pain. This results in lower extremity paralysis and total loss of bowel and bladder control. It is a procedure of last resort for intolerable intermittent lancinating pain from cancer or severe injury involving the lower extremities. Performed under general anesthesia, the surgeon must open up the spinal canal at the level of injury and several segments above it to gain access to the part of the cord needing removal; good pain relief is reportedly achieved in 80 percent of cases.

Brain Surgery

Brain surgery involves cutting the nerve tracks or pathways deep within the brain that are responsible for the transmission of pain. For example, mesencephalic tractotomy on one side may be effective in alleviating cancer pain of the opposite face, neck, or shoulder. Using stereotactic surgical methods, a computer-guided probe is inserted through a burr hole in the skull into the brain until it reaches the mesencephalic lateral spinothalamic tract. After verifying the proper probe position, a radiofrequency lesion is created in the tract that should produce loss of pain and temperature sensation on the opposite side of the body lasting six months or more.

SPINAL SURGERIES

Surgeons operate on the spine for a number of painful conditions including cervical, thoracic, lumbar, and lumbosacral intervertebral disc removal; spine fractures and other spine injuries; spinal synovial or ganglion cysts; spinal cord herniation syndromes; congenital deformities of the spine; syringomyelia (a disease of the spinal cord characterized by the development of cavities and destruction of nerve cells); vertebral hemangiomas (blood vessel tumors), nonmalignant nerve cell tumors, malignant nerve cell tumors (including astrocytoma, olgiodendroglioma, ependymoma, and ganglioglioma), spinal chondrosarcomas, other spine tumors; and spinal stenosis (narrowing of the space in the spinal column that the spinal cord goes through, compressing the cord). Many of these conditions involve very specific lesions or problems that can be surgically corrected.

Others involve less specific injuries and chronic conditions for which the success rate of surgery is much lower. Correct diagnosis is therefore essential. Magnetic resonance imaging (MRI) is often effective in detecting such conditions without invasive testing.

Decompression and Spinal Fusion

The vertebral bones form the spine by sitting on top of one another similar to well-matched building blocks. In between each vertebral bone is a cartilaginous fibrous cushion or disc that is filled with a gelatinous fluid; this fluid-filled vertebral disc acts as a shock absorber and also allows for flexibility in the spine. With time and aging, and sometimes trauma, bone spurs can form off of the vertebral bones. The vertebral disks themselves can wear out, collapse, and exude their gelatinous fluid, which then presses on nerves as they emerge from the spinal column. This causes pain, numbness, and sometimes weakness, leading to loss of function. Although physical therapy, exercises, and pain medications are the mainstay of treatment and can provide significant relief, surgery may be necessary if pain and disability continue. The surgery involves cutting open the back, removing the disc to decompress the nerves, and then permanently fixing, connecting, or fusing the vertebral bones to one another. This, of course, reduces the flexibility of the spine and its shock-absorber capacity, especially if several disks are involved and spinal fusion must be done at several different levels. Although this procedure may significantly reduce pain and disability (as it did for Jackie and Joan), many people continue to have pain following surgery (as did Bob).

Spinal Endoscopy

Spinal endoscopy is a new technique now in its experimental stages that may prove quite useful in the diagnosis and treatment of painful spinal problems. Although radiologic techniques such as CT and MRI scans are useful in detecting spinal problems, many instances occur in which scans are normal and yet the person still has pain. Spinal endoscopy may provide useful information in such cases because it allows the surgeon to visually examine the problem through a small, thin, lighted tube. Furthermore, procedures conducted through the endoscope may make it possible to treat certain conditions without requiring a major operation.

In some areas of the United States, endoscopic removal of herniated vertebral discs is being done as an outpatient procedure, which frequently allows patients to feel relief immediately after the thirty-minute operation. During this procedure, called lumbar endoscopic discectomy, an anesthesiologist provides intravenous sedation while the surgeon applies additional local anesthesia to the skin of the back over the affected vertebrae. With the help of X-ray guidance, a specially designed probe with a diameter of less than one-eighth inch is inserted through a tiny incision in the skin of the back and into the herniated or bulging disc space. A portion of the nuclear material near the herniation is then removed with a laser, suction, or other mechanical means, thereby lowering the pressure that the bulging disc is applying to surrounding nerves. The rest of the disc is left intact. The Western Neurosurgical Clinic in the San Francisco Bay area is one of many such places now performing this exciting new procedure <http://www.drschiffer.com/>. The procedure is now also done at the Barrow Neurological Institute of St. Joseph's Hospital and Medical Center in Phoenix, Arizona (visit <http://www.cdickmanmd.com/publicat/endsxltr.htm>) and at the La Jolla Spine Institute (visit <http://www.lajollaspine.com/PatientCare_Minimally Invasive.html>).

Rehabilitation

Physical therapy is extremely important after any type of surgery for chronic pain, whether this involves the back, hip, knee, or other body part. Rehabilitation includes the use of assistive devices at home to improve ambulation during convalescence and weight reduction to relieve stress on weight-bearing joints if involved. This is particularly true following any kind of spinal surgery.

Pain following surgery, however, can interfere with rehabilitation. Pain contributes to perioperative stress, increased catecholamine levels, blood clot formation, vasoconstriction, and immune suppression, all of which may interfere with tissue healing.[3] Furthermore, good pain control enables patients to participate more fully in their rehabilitation program, thus helping them recover more quickly and avoid many of the complications of surgery. Successful surgery always requires aggressive rehabilitation and adequate perioperative pain control.

NEGATIVE CONSEQUENCES OF SURGERY

Not only can surgical procedures be ineffective, they may also result in disastrous consequences. For example, surgery may destroy the pathways necessary to control pain through other sensory-input treatment methods (such as transcutaneous electrical nerve stimulation or implantable nerve stimulators). Pain may continue or become worse as a result of scars or neuromas that form as a result of the surgical procedure. Finally, pain may persist because it has become wired into the central nervous system and now exists independent of peripheral nerve inputs. In such cases, severing peripheral nerves or even the spinal cord produces little pain relief. In other cases, although temporary pain relief is achieved, pain returns after awhile. If loss of strength or paralysis has resulted from the surgery, then not only must the person cope with loss of function but also with the return of the pain.

TRANSCUTANEOUS ELECTRICAL NERVE STIMULATION

Of all the electrical therapies currently available, transcutaneous electrical nerve stimulation (TENS) is the closest to becoming universally adopted as a mainstream treatment for chronic pain. Recall the benefits that Bob and Joan received from their TENS units. TENS can be used for any type of localized physical pain, although it is most commonly advocated for arthritis, sciatica, neuralgia, and chronic back pain. It is sometimes used after knee, hip, or lower back surgery (usually in combination with other analgesics). TENS has also been used for dental pain, jaw muscle pain, cancer pain, angina pectoris, menstrual pain, migraine, carpal tunnel syndrome, repetitive strain injuries, nerve damage, musculoskeletal trauma, and shingles.

TENS is based on the gate-control theory of pain. In brief, this theory holds that the transmission of nerve impulses from peripheral parts of the body (arms, legs, or torso) to the spinal cord is controlled by a spinal gating mechanism located in the dorsal portion of the cord. This gate can open or close to allow or prevent nerve impulses from traveling up the spinal cord to the brain. This spinal gate is influenced by the amount of activity in large and small diameter nerve fibers; stimulation of large fibers tends to close the gate, whereas stimulation of smaller fibers tends to open the gate. TENS units produce electrical impulses that stimulate large nerve fibers, which close the spinal gate and thus prevent pain messages from smaller fibers from traveling up the spinal cord and reaching the brain where they are consciously perceived.

Modern TENS units are small portable devices containing a nine-volt battery that provides the electrical stimulation. Most units today have two channels that control a pair of electrodes placed over the painful body area. The patient, by turning a dial or switch, can vary the output frequency pulse width and intensity. The most commonly accepted theory of why TENS units work is that they modulate pain at the spinal cord level by closing the spinal gate (as discussed earlier). Other theories involve the stimulated release of natural substances such as endorphins that have analgesic properties. Pain relief with TENS is initially reported to be about 60 to 80 percent; with time, however, its effectiveness decreases to about 25 to 30 percent.

IMPLANTABLE NERVE STIMULATOR

Direct spinal cord stimulation has been around for about thirty years, but in the past five years its usefulness has been increasingly recognized by the medical community.[4] Previously performed only by neurosurgeons, it is now being used by anesthesiologists, orthopedic surgeons, and physiatrists. Computer-interactive programming is gaining popularity with today's ability to independently stimulate multiple arrays of electrodes in different areas of the spinal cord, nerve roots, and peripheral nerves. Research is showing this procedure to be effective, safe, and reliable. One study examined the effectiveness of spinal cord stimulation in the treatment of patients with chronic pain due to spinal cord injury, postherpetic neuralgia, failed back surgery, and brachial plexus injury. After an average twenty-one months of follow-up, three-quarters of patients had satisfactory improvement of pain.[5]

This implantable device works directly on the spinal cord or peripheral nerves by interfering with pain signals before they reach the brain. The most common method is spinal column nerve stimulation in which electrodes are placed in the epidural space and stimulate the part of the spinal cord where nerve tracts that transmit pain are located. This method does not destroy nerve tissue and is completely reversible. Such a device may provide good to excellent pain relief and improve daily function. Pain conditions most likely to respond to implantable neurostimulators are chronic low back pain following back surgery, painful neuropathies, and complex regional pain syndromes.[6] An example of a complex pain syndrome is reflex sympathetic dystrophy, a condition that occurs after an injury (such as a bone fracture) and is associated with extreme pain in a limb, loss of function, skin and temperature changes, swelling, and sensitivity to touch. Persons with back pain may have undergone multiple surgical procedures for disc herniation or injury of nerve roots, yet continue to experience chronic pain. Peripheral neuropathies often result from inflammation or degeneration of peripheral nerves due to diabetes or certain medications; pain is often experienced in the lower extremities and often involves both legs.

The spinal cord stimulator works through a small neurostimulation system that is surgically placed under the skin to send mild electrical impulses to the spinal cord. Electrical impulses are delivered through a medical wire (lead) that is surgically placed into the cord. These electrical impulses block the pain signals from reaching the brain. The peripheral nerve stimulator works in a similar way, but the medical wire is placed on the specific nerve causing the pain rather than near the spinal cord. Electrical impulses (felt as a tingling sensation) can be directed at the specific site where the pain is being felt. Makers of these devices claim they provide effective pain relief that can reduce or eliminate the need for repeat surgeries or pain medications.

At least two types of neurostimulators are available. The first is a totally implantable system that includes a pulse generator, programmer, and extension with leads. The second is a radiofrequency system that includes an external transmitter, antenna, implanted receiver, and leads. The primary difference between these neurostimulators is the location of the battery. In the totally implantable system, the battery is placed completely beneath the skin. This system is controlled with an external programmer that can be adjusted by the patient or the doctor. In the radiofrequency system, the battery is worn outside the body and requires that the person wear an antenna on their skin over the site of the receiver. At the present time, most people using neurostimulators use the totally implantable system. More information on implantable nerve stimulators can be obtained by visiting the Medtronics Web site (the largest producer of these devices) at <http://www.medtronic.com/neuro/pain/about4.html>.

Despite their growing usefulness, implantable therapies are expensive and must be inserted by those with considerable expertise in this technique (an anesthesiologist, often in collaboration with a surgeon). Patients are usually given a trial of one week to see if the device is effective in relieving pain before completing the operation.

MOTOR CORTEX STIMULATION

This procedure is used for the treatment of central and peripheral types of deafferentation pain (where pain is disconnected from its peripheral source as seen in certain neuropathic pain syndromes). In one of the few studies examining this procedure, four patients with thalamic (central) pain and four patients with peripheral deafferentation pain had electrodes implanted in their interhemispheric fissures to treat lower extremity pain. Six of eight patients experienced pain reduction from this procedure (two each with excellent, good, and fair relief). Two of the four cases of deafferentation pain had excellent results. They concluded that motor cortex stimulation was effective in relieving these types of pain.[7]

Electrical stimulation of the precentral gyrus is also emerging as a promising technique for pain control. PET scanning has been used to track these effects and uncover possible anatomical mechanisms.[8] In another study, thirty-two patients with refractory central and neuropathic pain of peripheral causes were treated with chronic stimulation of the motor cortex over a four-year period with an average follow-up of twenty-seven months.[9] Ten of thirteen patients with central pain and ten of twelve patients with neuropathic facial pain experienced substantial relief. One of three patients with postoperative pain syndrome was clearly improved. Satisfactory improvement was obtained for two other patients. No patients developed epileptic seizures, a concern whenever the brain is stimulated.

IMPLANTABLE DRUG DELIVERY SYSTEMS

These devices are most useful in patients with cancer-related pain who develop side effects to high doses of narcotic pain relievers. Even for selected patients with nonmalignant chronic pain, however, opioid infusion devices that deliver the drug directly to the spinal cord may be effective. Furthermore, patients with opioid-nonresponsive pain may benefit from the infusion of a combination of local anesthetics and opioid drugs (morphine, in particular).

A small pump is surgically placed just under the skin of the abdomen to deliver morphine directly to the intrathecal space surrounding the spinal cord. Delivered through a small surgically placed catheter, pain relievers such as morphine can be directed at specific sites along the spinal cord, controlling pain by using a much smaller dose than would be required if taken orally, thereby minimizing side effects. Further information about implantable drug delivery systems can be obtained by contacting the Medtronics Web site at <http://www.medtronic.com/neuro/pain/about4.html>.

INJECTIONS FOR THE RELIEF OF PAIN

Lumbar Facet Injections

For chronic low back pain, injections with local anesthetic (lidocaine) may be targeted at the lumbar vertebral joints called "facets." If pain is significantly relieved by two local injections to a lumbar facet, then radiofrequency destruction of the sensory nerves to the facet may bring lasting relief if physical therapy and exercise are not helpful.

Sacroiliac (SI) Joint Injections

For people who have one-sided low back pain that is worse upon sitting and can be elicited by pressure and forced movement of the SI joint, injection of the joint with local anesthetic may provide at least temporary relief and may identify the cause of the pain (long-term treatment involves physical therapy and exercise). Such injections are typically performed under X-ray fluoroscopy.

Epidural Injections

Epidural steroid injections (ESI), also used primarily for treating chronic low back pain, are thought to be particularly useful for relieving ongoing inflammation caused by a herniated disc. A small amount of steroid and local anesthetic is injected just outside of the covering of the spinal cord (called the dura) where nerve roots exit from the cord. Approximately 30 to 40 percent of low back pain patients experience relief of pain following medical or surgical treatment, whereas lumbar ESI is associated with a 25 to 75 percent significant relief of pain. Certain characteristics are known to predict a good response to ESI. These include relatively short duration of pain, under age fifty, no previous back surgery, radicular pattern to the pain (e.g., pain follows the known anatomic pathway of nerves), nerve root irritation, and low emotional reaction to the pain.

Complications to epidural injections (especially when steroids are combined with local anesthetic) include hypotension (drop in blood pressure), intravascular injection (injection into blood vessel, rather than around spinal cord), motor paralysis, cessation of respiration (for high epidural, subarachnoid, or subdural injections), and spinal headache due to puncture of the dura and leakage of spinal fluid.

Epidural or intrathecal infusion of opioids, baclofen, or local anesthetics can produce excellent pain relief in some cases of diabetic neuropathy and other pain syndromes. Internalized drug systems (as previously noted) can provide long-term relief.

Joint Aspiration and Injection

For a person with a severe swollen and tender joint due to inflammatory arthritis, the physician may decide to aspirate fluid (withdraw through a needle) from the joint sack (bursa) to relieve the pain caused by the swelling. Unfortunately, the fluid often rapidly reaccumulates if the inflammation continues. For this reason, the doctor may inject a steroid preparation into the joint to relieve the inflammation and thereby prevent the reaccumulation of the fluid. The general rule is that no more than three injections of steroid into the joint at intervals of six months or longer should be given; otherwise, such injections can accelerate the destruction of joint cartilage. Another risk of joint aspiration and steroid injection is the seeding of bacteria into the joint during the procedure, resulting in joint infection that can lead to further joint damage and may even result in the infection spreading throughout the body through the blood stream (septicemia).

EXPERIMENTAL THERAPIES

New technologies are continuously appearing on the frontier of chronic pain therapies. These include gene therapy and surgical implantation of cells that produce natural pain relievers.

Gene Therapy

Scientists at the National Institute of Dental and Cranial Facial Research and the University of Pennsylvania in Philadelphia are seeking to relieve chronic pain by injecting pain-relieving genes directly into the tissue surrounding the spinal cord.[10] A study involving rats demonstrated that injecting a gene that increases the production of beta-endorphins was successful in relieving pain. Researchers were able to show that connective tissue surrounding the spinal cord readily took up the injected genes. This was accomplished by using a virus to deliver the beta-endorphin gene to the tissues surrounding the spinal cord. The protective sheath around the spinal cord "soaked up" the virus, which did not infect the brain or spinal cord. Within twenty-four hours of injection, the connective tissues began producing beta-endorphins until levels were ten times greater than normal (which is sufficient to produce pain relief). Scientists speculated that such advances would soon lead to new treatments for chronic pain in patients with spinal cord injury and those with disorders such as multiple sclerosis and Parkinson's disease.

Cell Implantation

Cytotherapeutics in Lincoln, Rhode Island, is currently conducting clinical trials on humans, having implanted cow adrenal cells at the base of the spine.[11] These cells continuously secrete natural pain-killers that help boost the body's own capacity to relieve pain.

SUMMARY AND CONCLUSIONS

Neurosurgical procedures resulting in permanent destruction of nerve tissue are options of last resort for those with terminal illness and unrelenting pain. In general, surgical therapies for relief of chronic pain should be considered only after less invasive approaches have been tried and proven unsuccessful. There are exceptions to this rule, particularly when a specific pain syndrome is diagnosed for which there is an effective surgical therapy. Spinal surgery for herniated vertebral discs, especially when performed using the new endoscopic procedures, falls into the latter category; however, even this type of surgery does not always provide optimal pain relief and return of function. Both transcutaneous and implantable electrical nerve stimulators are relatively noninvasive approaches that have been used widely and successfully to provide pain relief. Opioid infusion devices may bring pain relief with fewer side effects by delivering narcotic pain relievers to specific areas of the spinal cord. New surgical and other mechanical technologies are constantly being developed and tested, promising future therapies that are less invasive and more effective for the relief of chronic pain.

Chapter 13

Specific Disease Conditions

This chapter discusses the management of the five most common conditions that cause chronic pain: osteoarthritis, fibromyalgia, headache, chronic back problems, and cancer. These conditions are responsible for well over 90 percent of pain complaints in the United States.

OSTEOARTHRITIS

Recall from Chapter 1 that many persons over age forty have signs of beginning arthritis or rheumatism, and 70 percent of those over age sixty-five show X-ray evidence of osteoarthritis. The most frequent cause of pain in older adults is osteoarthritis of the shoulder, hip, knee, and hand joints, and 44 percent of older Americans experience pain related to it. The cause of pain in osteoarthritis is different from the cause of pain in conditions such as rheumatoid arthritis, which is largely due to inflammation. Osteoarthritis affects the cartilage that covers the ends of bones where they meet at joints. Cartilage helps to cushion the places where bones connect and facilitates the gliding of one bone over another, as seen most prominently in hip and shoulder joints. The wear and tear caused by constant use over many years results in erosion of joint cartilage, causing bone to come into direct contact with bone, resulting in increased friction, microscopic bone fractures, and significant pain. Osteoarthritis tends to increase with age, although persons involved in heavy physical labor or contact sports may develop it in certain joints when they are younger.

Drug Treatments

Most drug treatments for osteoarthritis seek to relieve pain and not inflammation, although inflammation may play a minor role. For this reason, the treatment of first choice for osteoarthritis is acetaminophen (Tylenol), a pain reliever, not an anti-inflammatory drug. At doses of up to 4,000 mg/day (two 500 mg Tylenol tablets four times per day), acetaminophen has been shown in persons with osteoarthritis to provide equal pain relief to doses of nonsteroidal anti-inflammatory drugs (NSAIDs) such as ibuprofen (Motrin) 1,200 to 2,400 mg/day or naproxen (Naprosyn) 750 mg/day.[1] If acetaminophen by itself at doses up to 4,000 mg/day is not effective, then addition of a NSAID should be considered. The toxicity and cost of NSAIDs, however, are cause for concern.

One study found that 20 to 30 percent of all hospitalizations and deaths due to peptic ulcer disease in persons over age sixty-five were related to NSAID use—particularly in those with a history of peptic ulcer disease, taking corticosteroids or anticoagulants, smokers, or moderate to heavy alcohol drinkers. Misoprostol (Cytotec) may help to prevent peptic ulcer disease in susceptible individuals. Reversible kidney failure is also a concern (occurring in 1 to 5 percent of those taking NSAIDs), particularly in persons over age sixty-five, those with a history of high blood pressure or congestive heart failure, and those using diuretics or antihypertensives. Except for low-dose aspirin (81 to 325 mg/day), no NSAID should be used in combination with other NSAIDs.

COX-2 inhibitors belong to a new class of NSAIDs associated with fewer side effects, in particular gastrointestinal side effects (and possibly fewer kidney effects as well, although this is less certain). Celebrex and Vioxx are the best known COX-2 inhibitors (see Chapter 9), although meloxicam (M-cam or Mobic) is the most recently FDA-approved drug in this class (available in 7.5 mg and 15 mg tablets taken once daily). COX-2 inhibitors are quickly replacing standard NSAIDs in the treatment of chronic pain, especially pain from arthritis. These drugs decrease both pain and inflammation and are therefore useful for both osteoarthritis and inflammatory types of arthritis. A recent comprehensive review of the use of COX-2 inhibitors in the treatment of osteoarthritis concluded that these drugs have the potential for significant benefit in selected and carefully monitored persons with this condition.[2]

Tricyclic antidepressants (TCAs) (which have an analgesic action independent of effects on improving mood) may influence pain by affecting levels of serotonin and norepinephrine in the brain. Because TCAs also have sedative properties, they may be helpful for treating sleep problems commonly associated with osteoarthritic pain. Doses are usually substantially below those necessary for antidepressant effects. Selective serotonin reuptake inhibitors (such as Prozac, Paxil, or Zoloft) are not as effective as TCAs (Elavil or Pamelor), although they may be used to treat the depression and anxiety that often accompany pain.

If oral pain relievers fail to help the pain or for some other reason cannot be taken, consider adding topical analgesics such as capsaicin or methylsalicylate cream. Capsaicin is derived from hot chili peppers and is thought to reduce pain by depleting substance P in tissues, which is one of the biological mediators of pain and inflammation. It is recommended that capsaicin cream be applied four times per day to the skin overlying painful joints or muscles (see Appendix II for more information).

If pain persists in a single joint and is severe, injection of corticosteroids into the joint, such as triamcinolone hexacetonide (20 mg for a knee joint), causes relief of pain in most cases, but typically does not last very long (one to four weeks). Injections should not be given more frequently than once every three months (particularly into the knee) due to damage to the joint caused by repeated injections. Joint fluid should also be sent to the laboratory to rule out infection or gout. If steroid injections (together with oral medication) fail to relieve pain and swelling in an osteoarthritic joint, then the person should be evaluated for a surgical procedure (such as a joint replacement).

If all of these fail to lessen pain, which remains severe and interferes with function, then narcotic pain relievers should be considered. The use of narcotic analgesics for pain control in patients with chronic moderate to severe arthritis is controversial. This is due to concern over long-term effectiveness, toxicity, development of tolerance, dependence, addiction, and abuse, as well as physician concern over scrutiny by regulatory agencies for long-term prescribing of opium-derived narcotics for noncancer pain.[3] However, experience with long-term treatment of cancer pain has demonstrated sustained relief without the development of tolerance, a need to increase the dose, or abuse.[4,5]

Nevertheless, these same experts caution that doctors should always be alert to signs of addiction, including loss of control over drug use (overconcern with obtaining drug, manipulation of health care system, seeking drugs from multiple providers), compulsive drug use (intense desire for the drug, increased dose without doctor's permission), and continued drug use despite harmful consequences (legal problems, family difficulties, and trouble at work). True addiction, however, must be distinguished from "pseudoaddiction," in which the threat of discontinuation of an effective medication results in anxiety and drug-seeking behavior (due to undertreatment of pain).[6]

Narcotic analgesics that have been used to control severe osteoarthritic pain include propoxyphene (Darvon or Darvocet-N), codeine, oxycodone with tylenol (Larked, Vacation, Percocet, Roxicet, Tylox), oxycodone with aspirin (Percodan), and tramadol (Ultram). These drugs may be used to control pain during flare-ups of disease; they are administered in addition to the usual doses of nonnarcotic analgesics. Comparison studies have shown that tramadol (Ultram) at 50 to 100 mg three times daily is more effective than propoxyphene 65 mg (Darvocet-N100) three times daily. The general recommendation is that the addition of narcotic analgesics to acetaminophen, aspirin, or NSAIDs to control flare-ups of osteoarthritis pain should not continue for more than fourteen days.

Some experts, however, argue that long-term use of low-dose codeine or oxycodone is appropriate in persons with rheumatic disease pain that has not responded to other therapies. This is particularly true, they emphasize, since long-term use of opioid analgesics is not associated with any irreversible damage to major organs such as the gastrointestinal tract or kidneys (both of which are affected by NSAIDs). Furthermore, the majority of elderly patients (70 percent) do not experience significant side effects when taking 30 to 60 mg/day of codeine equivalent, and a large proportion (40 percent) have no side effects even when taking 120 to 360 mg/day. Nevertheless, these experts agree that side effects should be carefully monitored, particularly cognitive impairment, sedation, and increased risk of falling. Many of the side effects are temporary (lasting one to two weeks), although some may be more resistant to treatment (such as constipation).

There is also the problem of tolerance. The development of tolerance is indicated by a need to increase the dose of narcotic to maintain the same level of pain relief. In people experiencing true pain, however, tolerance is significantly less likely to develop than in those taking these drugs for recreational use. Carefully designed animal experiments support this statement. Tolerance does not occur as readily in animals experiencing pain, suggesting that physical pain may either prevent or modulate the development of tolerance.[7] In fact, it may be unethical to withhold opioid medication from patients in significant pain (including those with rheumatic conditions) for whom no other treatments have been effective.[8,9]

There is one caveat, however. Patients with rheumatic pain seen in primary care settings (outpatient offices of general physicians) should be distinguished from those seen in chronic pain clinics. Patients referred to chronic pain programs typically have a heavy overlay of psychological problems, social problems, and sometimes litigation issues that complicate the chronic prescribing of narcotic analgesics. Treatment in chronic pain programs focuses on detoxifying the patient from excessive analgesic use, substituting narcotic drugs with less harmful and less addictive substances, and paying attention to psychological and social rehabilitation, with the ultimate goal of increasing function, not necessarily decreasing pain.[10] However, primary care clinics typically focus on treating the underlying disease, reducing pain, and implementing exercise and psychosocial treatments to improve adaptation. By reducing pain, the goal is to increase rehabilitation to regain function. Furthermore, patients seen in a primary care setting typically see one physician and have lower rates of psychopathology and substance abuse than do those patients seen in chronic pain clinics.

Nondrug Treatments

The effective treatment of chronic pain from osteoarthritis involves a multipronged approach that includes drug therapy, education, cognitive-behavioral therapy, aerobic exercise and resistance training, massage, heat and cold applications, relaxation, biofeedback or self-hypnosis, distraction techniques, and application of transcutaneous electrical nerve stimulation (TENS) (see Chapters 10, 11, and 12)

Education is the first nondrug therapy in persons with osteoarthritis. Simply attending a self-help class has been shown to reduce pain, decrease physician visits, and increase overall quality of life. Such classes are offered through local branches of the Arthritis Foundation. Simple monthly telephone calls by trained nonmedical personnel have been shown to improve pain control and ability to function.[11]

Physical therapy (PT) plays an important role in the rehabilitation of osteoarthritis patients. PT may involve learning how to use a cane or walker to help improve joint mobility and function. PT also involves exercise training to maintain or improve joint motion range, flexibility, and muscle strength. Conditioning exercises include participation in a walking program to reduce pain, to increase walking time, and to decrease drug use and functional disability. Low-impact aerobic exercises (such as aquatics or walking) are ideal for those with osteoarthritis (see local Arthritis Foundation for location of exercise programs). Exercise will also help to reduce weight and decrease the stress placed on the joints with walking or other weight-bearing activity.

Patients with osteoarthritic pain in a particular joint (such as the knee) and significant limitation of movement despite drug and nondrug therapies may be candidates for *surgical treatment*. Surgical treatment includes either osteotomy or total joint replacement. Osteotomy involves the removal of bone spurs that may be interfering with joint movement and causing pain. This procedure is often performed on younger patients with plenty of motivation for rehabilitation. Total joint reconstruction is performed for pain relief and functional improvement. The quality of the surgical outcome depends on several factors, including the timing of surgery in relationship to the severity of joint disease, the quality of the surgeon, the patient's preoperative status, the quality of peri- and postoperative management, and the quality of the rehabilitation program.

If a person is not a candidate for joint surgery, several alternatives exist. These include closed-needle joint irrigation, arthroscopic lavage, and injection of hyaluronan. Closed-needle tidal joint irrigation involves irrigation of the joint with saline solution. Arthroscopic lavage, with or without debridement, is performed if the history and exam suggest internal derangements of cartilage or surrounding ligaments. Intra-articular injection of hyaluronan may also be attempted. Hyaluronan is a compound that binds proteoglycan molecules to form macromolecular aggregates inside the joint that act as a cushion and may reduce pain.

FIBROMYALGIA

Mary is a forty-one-year-old divorced bank teller who saw her primary care physician for chronic pain in her neck, back, pelvis, and upper legs. She reported having this problem for over ten years, and that it came on gradually during the early years of her first marriage when she was raising her three small children. At the time of the visit, Mary was taking a combination of a muscle relaxant (Flexeril, 10 mg three times per day), a narcotic analgesic (Darvocet N-100, four times per day), and a sleeping medication (Ambien, 10 mg at bedtime), but was not receiving much relief from the chronic pain which was beginning to affect her job performance. She was also becoming quite depressed and discouraged over her health condition.

A careful physical examination and blood evaluation were generally unremarkable, with the exception of several points of extreme tenderness when the doctor pressed his fingers down at certain places on her shoulders and lower back. A diagnosis of fibromyalgia was made, and Mary was instructed to begin to slowly cut back on her Darvocet dose. At the same time, the doctor prescribed two additional medications, Vioxx, 25 mg/day (for inflammation), and the antidepressant nortriptyline, 25 to 50 mg/day (for her depression and pain). He also referred her for physical therapy three times per week to help start an exercise regimen, and arranged to have her see a pastoral counselor to teach relaxation techniques and to help resolve some of the personal problems with which she was struggling.

Fibromyalgia is a difficult condition to have because there is no diagnostic test that definitively proves the diagnosis, and most other routine diagnostic tests are normal. Consequently, many doctors have concluded that this is a psychosomatic illness (symptoms that result from psychological causes, not physical ones). However, there is growing consensus that this disease does have a biological or medical cause, and is not psychosomatic.[12]

According to the American College of Rheumatology (ACR), fibromyalgia is an inflammatory rheumatic condition characterized by widespread muscle pain and spasm, chronic fatigue, difficulty sleeping, and, especially, specific muscle areas that are extremely tender when pressure is applied (called trigger points).[13] The ACR's diagnostic criteria for fibromyalgia are the following (*all* must be present): (1) widespread pain of at least three months duration; (2) pain on the right and left sides of the body, pain above and below the waist, and pain along the spine or anterior chest; (3) pain when a nine-pound force is applied with the fingers to at least eleven of the following eighteen sites: back of the head, low posterior neck, upper back above the shoulder blades, upper back below the shoulder blades, second rib near middle of anterior chest, just above the elbow, the outer part of the buttocks, the hip, and the knee (the right and left sides of the body are considered for each of these nine points, which makes eighteen trigger points). As with all chronic pain conditions, the symptoms of this disorder tend to improve and worsen spontaneously over time, and psychological or social stress can lead to flare-ups.

Drug Treatments

For those with only mild symptoms, simply knowing the diagnosis and recognizing it as a legitimate physical condition may be sufficient. It is particularly important for these individuals to develop and maintain a regular exercise regimen that will keep muscles limber and conditioned. Acetaminophen (1,000 mg up to four times per day) may be used to control minor pain symptoms and facilitate sleep at night. If this is not effective, a low dose of one of the newer NSAIDs (such as Vioxx or Celebrex) may help to relieve symptoms. NSAIDs, however, may have significant side effects (see Chapter 9).

Persons with more severe symptoms of fibromyalgia often require a more extensive therapeutic plan. This may include psychotherapy, medication, physical therapy, and even massage or possibly acupuncture (see Chapter 11). Of particular importance, however, is the doctor/patient relationship. Patients need to feel that their doctor takes their pain complaints seriously and is willing to work with them to help obtain relief. Other health conditions are frequently associated with fibromyalgia and require attention, including migraine headache, chronic fatigue, irritable bowel syndrome, depression, and rest-less leg syndrome.

In addition to analgesics such as acetaminophen and NSAIDs, anti-depressants are frequently prescribed for fibromyalgia. Although tri-cyclic antidepressants (such as Elavil or Pamelor) tend to be more helpful than the newer selective serotonin reuptake inhibitors (like Prozac or Zoloft), sometimes combinations of these drugs can reduce associated depression and produce mild to moderate relief of pain symptoms as well. Controlled studies show that approximately one-third to one-half of patients respond to this treatment. One study found that 25 mg of Elavil and 20 mg of Prozac when used together was twice as effective as when used separately. Elavil should be taken about two or three hours before bedtime, and doses may start as low as 10 mg. Older adults, however, should be very cautious when using this drug given its side effects. Some persons are extremely sensitive to tricyclic antidepressants and may need to be started on very low doses that are slowly increased. For example, doxepin (Sinequan) elixir may need to be started as low as one drop (less than 1 mg) and slowly increased. If depression is also present, then doses of the anti-depressant should be increased to standard therapeutic levels.

Studies have also shown that cyclobenzaprine (Flexeril) (which has a chemical structure similar to the antidepressant Elavil) may help to reduce symptoms in patients with fibromyalgia, which is con-sistent with my clinical experience. This drug, however, can be very sedating and should be used cautiously when driving or operating machinery. Side effects may be similar to those of Elavil (see Appen-dix II).

Narcotic analgesics may be used to treat pain in persons with fibromyalgia. These should be reserved only for those with severe pain that is causing significant functional impairment *and* for whom other therapies have either been ineffective or cannot be tolerated. The recommended narcotic analgesics in such cases are either slow-release oxycodone (Roxicodone) or morphine sulfate (Duramorph). Any person for whom these medications are prescribed should be in-formed about the possibility of dependence and then carefully moni-tored for medication misuse. As with any narcotic, the body may ac-commodate to the pain-relieving effects of the drug, requiring that the dose be increased to maintain relief of symptoms (development of tolerance). With increasing dose, however, comes increasing side effects that may not be easily adjusted to, such as severe constipation and cognitive or mental status changes.

Nondrug Treatments

Studies have shown that physical exercise is associated with a reduction of pain and improvement of sleep in persons with fibromyalgia. Aerobic and muscle strengthening exercises are particularly helpful. Because it is difficult for many people to maintain an exercise regimen, it is important to provide regular encouragement of this activity and perhaps even suggest involvement in an exercise group to improve compliance. Exercise tends to increase muscle flexibility and reduce muscle tension, as well as decrease stress level.

In some cases, acupuncture may help. A recent meta-analysis of research studies on the effectiveness of acupuncture in fibromyalgia confirmed its effectiveness when used in combination with more traditional therapies.[14] The frequency of treatments typically ranges from once weekly to once every ten to twelve weeks. Information on how to locate an acupuncturist can be obtained by logging onto the Web site <http://www.medicalacupuncture.org>.

Cognitive-behavioral therapy is frequently beneficial to those who must cope with difficulties in social relationships and work environments because of their symptoms (see Chapter 10). Social isolation and feelings of inadequacy and low self-esteem are prevalent in this condition and must be addressed in any comprehensive treatment program. Relaxation therapies may also be used effectively to relieve muscle tension and spasms that cause pain and increase inflammation. Finally, hypnosis has been used effectively to improve functioning and reduce pain. Thus, a combination of acetaminophen, NSAID therapy if necessary, and a tricyclic antidepressant, together with an exercise regimen, and cognitive-behavioral and relaxation therapy may help patients with fibromyalgia to lead functional, meaningful lives. Spiritual strategies can often add significant benefits on top of those obtained through use of traditional therapies (see Chapter 14).

HEADACHE

Sarah is a seventy-three-year-old married woman who sought treatment for chronic headaches experienced over the past forty years. These headaches worsened significantly after the death of an adult son during a boating accident with her husband about thirty years ago. The headaches were described as constant and severe, located toward the back of her head. Sometimes they would occur on one side of the head, but most of the time on both sides. The headaches lasted for hours, sometimes an entire morning or even the entire day. She had seen many doctors for this condition, without obtaining significant relief.

She was now taking five Fiorinal tablets each day and was still having painful headaches daily (a single Fiorinal tablet is a combination of the barbiturate butalbital 50 mg, aspirin 325 mg, and caffeine 40 mg). In addition, she was experiencing increasing symptoms of depression and irritability, and her blood pressure had increased lately. She indicated that in the mornings she had several large cups of coffee, which seemed to help ease her headaches, especially if she woke up with them.

On evaluation, Sarah was diagnosed with chronic tension headaches (with perhaps an element of migraine), depression, caffeine-induced blood pressure elevation, and barbiturate dependence. The treatment team did not think she was "addicted" to the Fiorinal, since she had not increased her dose during the past two years and was not actively seeking the drug from multiple physicians—although admittedly she was close to being addicted.

Sarah was treated by slowly reducing the Fiorinal dose over a period of about three months and starting two extra-strength Tylenol (500 mg tablets) four times per day. She was instructed to replace her heavy coffee intake with decaffeinated coffee and avoid caffeinated beverages in the future. Sarah was also started on the TCA nortriptyline (Pamelor) at 10 mg at night, which was gradually increased over a month to achieve a therapeutic blood level that required 50 mg/day. Her headaches persisted (although did not noticeably worsen), so she was started on the beta-blocker Inderal, which helped to control the frequency of the headaches.

Studies show that the chronic use of pain medications such as Fiorinal for more than two consecutive days a week results in worse headaches and greater dependence on the medication. These are called analgesic rebound headaches. When tapered off medication, the majority of patients actually experience a greater than 50 percent *reduction* in the frequency and severity of headache.[15]

At the same time as medication changes were being instituted, Sarah was referred along with her husband for counseling. Behavioral treatments (biofeedback, guided imagery, and progressive relaxation) were also initiated. Using this multipronged approach, the treatment team was able to treat Sarah's headaches and depression, improve her family relationships and stress level, and eliminate the Fiorinal dependence.

Management strategies for any particular headache depend on the type of headache. Determining the correct diagnosis, then, becomes crucial for effective management. There are four basic types of headaches: migraine without aura, migraine with aura, tension headache, and cluster headache. Below are definitions for each developed by the International Headache Society.[16]

- *Migraine* without *aura*. At least five attacks fulfilling all of the following four criteria:
    1. Headaches last four to seventy-two hours (with or without treatment).
    2. Headaches have at least two of the following characteristics: unilateral location (pain on one side of the head), pulsating quality, moderate or severe intensity prohibiting daily activities, or aggravated by walking up stairs or similar routine physical activity.
    3. During the headache, at least one of the following symptoms occurs: nausea, vomiting, photophobia (pain worse in the presence of bright lights), or phonophobia (pain worse in the presence of loud sounds).
    4. No evidence of another medical cause for the symptoms.
- *Migraine* with *aura*. At least two attacks that include at least three of the following characteristics (and no other medical cause exists for the symptoms):

1. One or more fully reversible aura symptoms indicating brain dysfunction (visual scintilations, sparks, jagged lines, or other sensory phenomena).
2. At least one symptom develops gradually over more than four minutes or two or more symptoms occur one right after the other.
3. No single aura symptom lasts for more than one hour.
4. Headache follows the aura within one hour (headache may also begin before or at the same time as the aura).

- *Episodic tension-type headache.* There have been at least ten previous headache episodes that fulfill all the following criteria (if number of days with such headaches are greater than fifteen per month, then called *chronic tension headache*):
  1. Headaches last from thirty minutes to several days.
  2. Headaches are associated with at least two of the following characteristics: pressing/tightening (nonpulsating) quality, mild or moderate intensity (does not prevent activities), located on both sides of the head, or not aggravated by walking up stairs or similar routine physical activity.
  3. Nausea, vomiting (anorexia may occur), photophobia, or phonophobia are not present.
- *Cluster headache.* There have been at least five attacks fulfilling all of the following criteria:
  1. Severe one-sided pain around the eye and/or temple area lasting from 15 to 180 minutes untreated.
  2. Headache is associated with one or more of the following signs on the side of the pain: redness of the eye, tearing, nasal congestion, runny nose, forehead and facial sweating, pinpoint pupil, droopy eyelid, or swollen eyelid.
  3. Frequency of attacks is anywhere from one every other day to eight per day.

Treatment for Migraines (with or without Aura)

There are basically two categories of treatment: nondrug and drug. Nondrug interventions include patient education and behavioral methods. Patient education provides information about maintaining regular habits and avoiding headache triggers (alcohol, certain foods, stressful situations, etc.). Behavioral methods, which are often the treatment of choice for pregnant women, children, and adolescents, include cognitive-behavioral therapy, relaxation techniques, and biofeedback. Drug treatments fall into two categories: therapy for individual attacks (acute) and therapy to reduce the frequency, duration, and severity of attacks (prophylactic).

Drugs used in acute therapy must work quickly to stop the headache before it reaches its full severity. These drugs can be taken as a pill or as a nasal spray, or can be injected under the skin (subcutaneously). Medications that can be taken orally in tablet form at the start of an attack include, from weakest to strongest: acetaminophen and aspirin (Excedrin Migraine), nonsteroidal anti-inflammatory drugs (Naprosyn), ergotamine-type medications (cafergot or Wigraine), drug combinations (Midrin, which is a combination of acetaminophen, a mild sedative, and blood vessel constrictor), sumatriptan (Imitrex) or zolmitriptan (Zomig), barbiturate combinations (Fioricet or Fiorinal), and narcotics (Percodan or Percocet).

Sumatriptan and related drugs have contributed enormously to the treatment of migraine headache. They are highly effective in reducing or eliminating the pain, and can be administered by many different routes (orally, nasally, or by subcutaneous injection). Unfortunately, the "triptans" are quite expensive. In the long run, however, they may actually save money because they help to reduce the frequency of emergency-room and doctor visits. The biggest concern with these drugs, however, is they produce vasoconstriction in all blood vessels of the body, including the coronary arteries and cerebral arteries. Consequently, side effects include tightness of chest, paresthesias, and flushing, and the drug is contraindicated in patients with coronary artery disease, history of stroke, or peripheral vascular disease. Sumatriptan is available in 25 and 50 mg tablets, and 50 mg is the recommended single dose, with up to 300 mg per day if necessary (but no more).

Other triptans now available besides sumatriptan include zolmitriptan (Zomig). Zomig is available in 2.5 and 5 mg tablets, with a recommended dose of 2.5 mg to a maximum total dose of 10 mg per day. Naratriptan (Amerge) is another triptan and is available in 1 and 2.5 mg tablets, with a recommended dose of 2.5 mg to a maximum total of 5 mg per day. Rizatriptan (Maxalt), the fastest acting of the oral triptans, is available in 5 and 10 mg tablets, with a recommended dose of 10 mg per day. Only the 5 mg dose of rizatriptan should be used by persons also taking Inderal for prophylaxis.

Nausea and vomiting during a migraine may prevent pill taking, although oral hydroxyzine (Vistaril or Atarax 10, 25, or 50 mg) or metoclopramide (Reglan 10 mg) may reduce nausea. If oral medications cannot be taken, rectal suppositories such as Phenergan or Compazine may help. Since these latter medications can cause severe, prolonged spasm of the neck muscles, called dystonia or torticollis, they should be used cautiously. Phenergan or Compazine, when taken together with a 50 mg Indocin (an NSAID) suppository, is reported to successfully relieve headache in about 70 percent of cases. Cafergot suppositories may also effectively abort a migraine attack, although to prevent the development of nausea and vomiting it is important to start with only one-quarter to one-third of a suppository. This can be repeated as needed about every twenty or thirty minutes until the headache pain goes away.

An alternative to suppositories are nasal sprays, which work faster than tablets. Sumatriptan (Imitrex), dihydroergotamine (Migranal), and butorphanol (Stadol NS) are all available in this form. For Imitrex, the usual dose is 20 mg sprayed into one nostril. This dose may be repeated only once within any given twenty-four-hour period. Migranal and Stadol are more difficult to use and may have more side effects than Imitrex.

Agents that are administered by subcutaneous or intramuscular injection include the ergotamine preparation, DHE-45, that can be given as a 1 mg dose initially and then repeated after one hour if necessary. The onset of action, however, is slow and the drug is often associated with significant nausea. Sumatriptan (Imitrex) can be given as a 6 mg dose subcutaneously (the most effective way of delivering the drug) but the recurrence rate of headache is high. This dose also may be repeated only one time within a twenty-four-hour period.

Narcotics may be administered orally, subcutaneously, or intramuscularly and are often highly effective in relieving the pain of migraine. Other treatment options should be utilized first to stop the headache (such as sumatriptan), rather than simply reducing the headache pain with a narcotic drug.

In order to decrease the frequency, duration, and severity of migraine attacks, prophylaxis therapy should be considered. This means taking a medication on a daily basis to prevent the onset of migraine headaches. Recall that Penny in Chapter 4 experienced relief from severe recurrent migraine headaches when her doctors placed her on a regular dose of Inderal. Prophylaxis is indicated if a person must take acute medicine for headache two or more days per week (this is in order to prevent the problem of rebound headache, as Sarah experienced taking five Fiorinal per day). Prophylactic therapy is also appropriate if acute medication for migraine is ineffective or if migraine attacks cause serious disability or other health problems. Prophylactic medications include beta-blockers (Inderal), calcium channel agents (Calan SR), heterocyclic antidepressants (nortriptyline or amitriptyline), and anticonvulsants (such as Depakote or Neurontin).

The particular medication chosen for prophylactic therapy should be selected based on the other mental or physical health conditions of the patient. For example, someone with depression or anxiety might benefit most from an antidepressant. The person with migraine and bipolar disorder or seizure disorder should take Depakote or Neurontin. Calan SR would be best for someone with Raynaud's phenomenon, whereas a beta-blocker such as Inderal might be prescribed for the person with mitral valve prolapse.

Treatment for Tension Headaches

Mild tension headaches are usually treated by taking over-the-counter treatments such as acetaminophen or aspirin. For more severe headaches, NSAIDs such as Naprosyn or Motrin may be effective. Persons with moderate to severe tension headaches who also have a history of migraine may receive benefit from sumatriptan and related drugs. Remember, however, that medications taken for the acute headache (especially opiates or barbiturates) should be limited to no more than two days per week to avoid analgesic rebound headaches (as Sarah had). If tension headaches are frequent and severe, then they can be prevented by the same drugs used for prophylaxis in migraine. Occasionally, use of muscle relaxants such as metaxalone (Skelaxin) or carisoprodol (Soma) may help. Nondrug therapies should always be instituted in persons with frequent and severe tension headaches, since stress or an ongoing psychosocial problem is often the cause or at least a contributor.

Treatment of Cluster Headaches

Cluster headaches are uncommon and often misdiagnosed. These headaches may be so severe that suicide is contemplated (the headache that Penny describes in Chapter 4 may actually have been a cluster headache misdiagnosed as a migraine). The pain in a cluster headache usually increases very rapidly to a maximum pain intensity within fifteen minutes. During such an attack, the most effective treatment is inhalation of 100 percent oxygen at greater than 7 liters/minute, which will quickly abort the attack. Persons who experience headaches at night may keep an oxygen container next to their bedside. Those experiencing attacks during the day may carry a small portable oxygen tank with them to work or in the car. Alternatively, a 6 mg subcutaneous injection of sumatriptan may help to relieve the pain. Unfortunately, however, use of sumatriptan is discouraged in older persons (particularly men over age forty), those who smoke, have high blood pressure, or have other risk factors for coronary artery disease or stroke.

Some people with cluster headaches may have several per day, limiting the effectiveness of sumatriptan injections, which may be given only twice per twenty-four-hour period. As an alternative to sumatriptan, butorphanol administered by nasal inhalation (Stadol NS) may be rapidly effective (although dosing needs to be monitored due to the potential for misuse of this medication). Prophylactic therapy should be considered for persons with frequent and severe episodes of cluster headache. A seven- to ten-day course of prednisone at 60 to 80 mg per day given at the onset may help to abort the headache series. A number of other prophylactic therapies such as the calcium channel blocker Calan SR (at a dose of up to 480 mg/day), lithium, or the anticonvulsant Depakote may also be effective in preventing attacks.

CHRONIC BACK PAIN

The treatment of chronic back pain requires a focus on rehabilitation. After careful evaluation of the cause of back pain, which includes a medical history, physical examination, and review of the X rays, a diagnosis is made. The diagnosis is important because this will help determine prognosis and direct the treatment plan. A prognosis is a prediction of the likely long-term course of a condition.

Managing chronic low back pain typically involves a team of experts who work together toward two goals: relief of pain and improvement of functioning. Physical therapists are an important part of this team, and they assist by designing passive and active programs for physical reconditioning. Passive treatments involve ultrasound, heat, and cold. Active treatments involve a graded exercise program specially designed to minimize further injury and to maximize muscle strength and functioning. Teaching body mechanics and back care are important parts of the treatment plan. Mental health specialists may also be involved to help the patient cope better with the pain and to follow the prescribed medication and exercise regimen.

Medications are not discussed here because they are similar to those previously discussed for osteoarthritis. Besides medications, other treatment modalities are frequently used with success, including biofeedback, transcutaneous electrical nerve stimulation, and, more recently, implantable spinal cord stimulation. Occasionally, injection of spinal column facets or epidural steroid injection is helpful, and at times, referral to a neurosurgeon for a back operation becomes necessary. Transcutaneous nerve stimulation, spinal cord stimulation, and the newest forms of back surgery (including transcutaneous arthroscopic discectomy) are discussed in Chapter 12.

CANCER-RELATED PAIN

Many barriers exist to the adequate treatment of pain in people with cancer.[17] This is especially true for those living in nursing homes. One recent study found that 38 percent of a large random sample of nursing home patients with cancer experienced daily pain.[18] Despite this, 26 percent received no pain medication whatsoever. In that study, persons over the age of eighty-five and those in minority groups were least likely to receive pain medication. Only about half of all nursing home patients with pain who were candidates for narcotic pain relievers (according to the World Health Organization criteria) were actually receiving these drugs. Many doctors fail to treat pain adequately because they do not have sufficient experience or training in the management of cancer pain. There is inappropriate concern about the side effects of narcotic pain relievers and their addiction potential in the setting of terminal illness. A lower priority is given by doctors to pain control than to disease management (directed at amelioration or cure).

Barriers also exist from the cancer patient's side. There is underreporting of pain to doctors. There is noncompliance to narcotic drug therapy for fear of addiction or because of pressure by family members, friends, or caregivers. There are impediments in the health care system which make it difficult for those with cancer to receive the right pain medication at the right time. There are socioeconomic issues. Many of these barriers, both on the doctor's side and the patient's side, can be overcome by education.

The following recommendations are meant for people with cancer receiving palliative care.[19] Palliative care is the type of medical care that does not seek to cure the disease but rather to maximize comfort, quality of life, and level of functioning.

The use of narcotic analgesics (opium-derived pain relievers) for cancer pain is strongly endorsed by almost all national and international experts.[20] According to World Health Organization (WHO) criteria,[21] mild to moderate pain should be treated with codeine, tramadol (Ultram), or propoxyphene (Darvon or Darvocet). Moderate to severe pain should be treated with morphine, methadone, oxycodone, buprenorphine, hydromorphone, fentanyl, or even heroin if no other opiate is effective. One thing is certain: WHO criteria indicate that narcotic pain relievers should be the mainstay of therapy for cancer-related pain. Despite this, nearly 40 percent of persons with cancer do not receive drugs according to these guidelines. WHO guidelines include methods of comprehensive assessment, drug selection, route selection, and drug dosing, as well as use of alternative opioids, treatment of side effects, and monitoring for effectiveness.[22]

Using WHO guidelines, approximately 80 to 90 percent of pain due to cancer can be treated effectively with narcotic analgesics taken orally in combination with adjuvant drugs, with good relief.[23] Admittedly, however, the remaining 10 to 20 percent of pain can be difficult to treat.[24]

Morphine

Morphine is the drug of first choice in hospices and palliative care units for chronic management of moderate to severe pain. This medicine provides effective pain relief, has relatively few side effects, is simple to administer, and is relatively inexpensive. The oral route is the preferred method of administration. The peak pain-relieving effect of oral morphine occurs twenty to ninety minutes after ingestion, and it continues to be effective for about four to six hours. Oral morphine should be given in a simple water solution or as a tablet. Older adults have a higher sensitivity to the drug because their bodies cannot metabolize it (break it down) as quickly. Younger persons, therefore, may require higher doses to achieve the same pain-relieving effect as in older adults.[25] The effective dose of oral morphine varies considerably among patients because of variability in pain severity, perception by patient, and individual differences in drug metabolism.

The typical dose ranges from 5 to 30 mg every four hours, although some persons may require higher doses. Slow-release oral morphine may be administered two or three times per day. Sometimes oral morphine may stop working. In that case, the doctor should consider changing to either the subcutaneous or epidural routes, which may be more effective in providing pain relief.[26] Morphine does not have a "ceiling effect." (The ceiling effect means that above a certain dose no further increases in dose will result in further pain relief. That is not true for oral morphine.[27] Only side effects limit dose.)

Side effects of morphine include the following.[28] Approximately 70 percent of cancer patients taking morphine experience nausea and vomiting. This problem tends to decrease with time, especially after taking the drug for about three weeks. Nausea and vomiting tend to be more frequent among persons who are able to walk about and be active compared to those confined to bed. Nausea and vomiting are the result of the effects of morphine on inner ear and balance centers in the brain (also called vestibular effects). Anticholinergic and antihistaminic drugs such as diphenhydramine (Benadryl) or hydroxyzine (Vistaril or Atarax) may help reduce nausea. If vomiting is a problem, consider domeperidone (Motilium), metoclopramide (Reglan), or cisapride (Propulsid), and if vomiting still persists, try haloperidol (Haldol). Slow-release oral morphine may cause less nausea and vomiting. If gastrointestinal symptoms continue to be a problem, however, morphine may be administered subcutaneously or via spinal catheter.

Constipation is present in approximately 50 percent of persons taking morphine, most frequently in the elderly. Constipation may also be due to reduced food and fiber intake, dehydration, or inactivity and deconditioning. Constipation can be managed with increased water intake and use of stimulant laxatives such as senna (Senokot), phenolphthalein (Ex-Lax), or cascara sagrada (BP-X, LB-X) if these are initiated as soon as morphine is started.

Sedation, lethargy, and extreme sleepiness can occur with the use of morphine. This effect is most problematic in the first twenty-four to seventy-two hours after starting morphine for the first time, and is dependent on the size of the dose. Once a person is on a stable dose, sedation does not appear to affect motor performance or even driving ability.[29] Family members should be educated that sleepiness or somnolence is only a temporary symptom and that pain control will be achieved with increasing alertness over time. To minimize sedation, short-acting oral morphine can be given every four hours to start with, and the dose gradually increased over time. If there is both persistent excessive sedation and poor pain control, an evaluation should be done for depression and other psychosocial issues which may be affecting the pain experience. Some patients with advanced cancer, however, are not able to achieve adequate pain control in the absence of sedation. The use of methylphenidate (Ritalin) may help to reduce sedation in such cases.

Dry mouth accompanies the use of morphine approximately 50 to 60 percent of the time. This may present as burning, ulceration, or soreness of the mouth, and can be accompanied by difficulty swallowing and even trouble speaking. Loss or change of taste may also occur. Dry mouth can be partially relieved by sipping water frequently, chewing gum, or sucking on hard candies.

Depression of respiratory rate is relatively rare, especially with oral morphine, although it can be serious and sometimes life threatening. This side effect is most prominent when patients first receive the drug. As the drug is taken over time, the effect of morphine on the rate of respiration decreases. In patients accustomed to taking morphine, only a large increase in dose will cause a reduction in breathing rate. Respiratory depression almost always occurs in the presence of deep sedation, which may be an early warning sign. If slowed breathing becomes a problem, the dose of morphine can be reduced or naloxone (0.2 mg every three minutes) can be administered, which will reverse the effect.

Another unpleasant side effect experienced by some patients is sweating (25 to 30 percent), which can be eliminated by either reducing or increasing the dose of morphine. Itching, although relatively rare, is another side effect that can be very disturbing. As with sweating, changing the morphine dose may reduce itching. The use of diphenhydramine (Benadryl) may also help, as will good skin care and use of topical anti-itch creams.

A number of side effects, while not evident early on, may emerge with long-term use of morphine. Hyperalgesia is an exaggerated pain response to a given stimulus, whether that stimulus is a painful or even a nonpainful sensory experience. This may occur because one of the metabolites or by-products of morphine antagonizes or counteracts the pain-relieving properties of morphine. If this side effect develops, a different opiate such as methadone or fentanyl should be tried (allowing the metabolites of morphine to clear out of the body); after awhile, the patient may be restarted on morphine. Myoclonus is the occurrence of sudden, brief involuntary movements caused by strong muscular contractions. It may be improved by switching from morphine to some other narcotic analgesic, such as methadone. Myoclonus may also be reduced by taking clonazepam (Klonopin) or diazepam (Valium).

Confusion or delirium is common in persons with advanced cancer. Morphine, however, can also contribute to this problem. Many other causes of delirium need to be ruled out first, including metabolic changes, infection, the spread of cancer to the brain, and effects of other drugs. Confusion may be improved by rotating narcotic analgesics (switching from morphine to methadone and, after awhile, back to morphine), increasing water intake (hydration), or stopping other drugs that may be causing delirium. In rare cases morphine may result in visual hallucinations, even in the absence of delirium or confusion. Again, narcotic analgesic rotation should be considered, and if the problem is serious, administration of antipsychotics for relief. Morphine, methadone, and oxycodone (Percodan or Percocet) may all have different side-effects, and intolerance to one drug may prompt switching to another with good results.

Drug Dosing

The goal in treating cancer pain is to achieve a balance between pain relief and side effects. Patients with continuous or frequently recurring cancer pain almost always respond best to fixed doses of an opioid drug given regularly. In other words, morphine should be prescribed every four to six hours, not simply on an as needed or PRN basis. Additional doses may also be needed for "breakthrough" pain. Breakthrough pain is temporary pain above and beyond that which the person normally experiences. Such pain may be caused by a voluntary action, such as pressing on a bone infiltrated with cancer that occurs against a background of adequately controlled pain on an already-established drug regimen.

The initial dose for someone who has never received narcotic pain relievers should be equivalent to about 5 to 10 mg of parenteral (intravenous, intramuscular, or subcutaneous) morphine or 15 to 30 mg of oral morphine every four hours. As-needed (PRN) doses for breakthrough pain are typically 5 to 15 percent of the total daily dose. The minimal interval for oral dosing is every two hours but can be as short as ten to fifteen minutes if intravenous morphine is being used. If pain is not relieved, the daily dose may be increased by 30 to 50 percent of the current daily dose, or by the equivalent to the total amount of PRN medication given in the past twenty-four hours. If pain relief is not sufficient or side effects are intolerable, it may be necessary to switch to a different drug. When "rotating" among different opiates, the dose should be reduced by 30 to 50 percent for the new drug (or by 90 percent, if switching to methadone). As previously noted, opiates such as morphine have no maximum dose or ceiling effect, and increasing the dose will result in increased pain relief. In some patients, as noted earlier, adequate pain relief is not possible before side effects limit the dose.

Adjuvant Drugs

Adjuvant drugs are prescribed for a primary condition other than pain but also provide pain relief for some painful conditions. They are useful after nonopioid and opioid drugs have been tried at their maximum tolerable doses. Adjuvant drugs include amitriptyline (Elavil) at a dose of 10 mg to 75 mg/day, and anticonvulsants such as Depakote 200 mg to 800 mg twice daily, Tegretol 200 mg to 400 mg twice daily, and Neurontin 100 mg to 1,200 mg three times daily. Neurontin (gabapentin) doses may need to be pushed up as high as 4,000 to 5,000 mg daily to get adequate relief;[30] at those doses, however, sedation can be a real problem. In some cases, antiarrhythmic drugs such as mexiletine 50 to 200 mg three times daily may be helpful when antidepressants and anticonvulstants are not effective. Corticosteroids such as dexamethasone 8 mg/day may be used to improve pain, anorexia, nausea, and fatigue. Bisphosphonates, radiopharmaceutical drugs, and calcitonin have been used effectively for malignant bone pain. Anticholinergics, octreotide, and corticosteroids may help to reduce pain and vomiting caused by bowel obstruction.

Anesthetic Techniques

Sometimes pain from cancer is so severe that neither pills nor injections will provide relief. In that case, spinal administration of drugs (into the epidural or subarachnoid space surrounding the spine or brain) may be effective. Other alternatives include destruction of nerve tissue such as a coeliac plexus block (for cancers of the stomach or pancreas), subarachnoid neurolysis (chemicals placed on nerve roots just as they exit the spinal cord or brainstem to destroy nerves irreversibly), or cordotomy (spinal cord is partially cut to interrupt nerve pathways to brain) (see Chapter 12). The conditions necessary for procedures that destroy nerve tissue are an accurate diagnosis of the cause of pain, a condition that will respond to the technique, a risk-benefit ratio acceptable to the patient, and failure of oral, intramuscular, and intravenous analgesics (and local anesthetic blocks).

Other Treatments

Radiation therapy and even palliative chemotherapy can be used for the sole purpose of reducing pain, not reversing the cancer. For example, chemotherapeutic agents such as gemcitabine and mitoxantrone have been approved by the FDA for treatment of pain in patients with pancreatic or prostate cancer.

Nondrug treatments include counterirritation techniques such as rubbing a painful body part with heat or ice, acupuncture, and transcutaneous or implantable nerve stimulators. Physiotherapy helps to maintain mobility, muscle flexibility, muscle tone, and ability to function. Occupational therapy teaches how a person can regain a particular function needed for independence without eliciting pain. Surgery may be necessary to provide stabilization of the spine or a long bone such as the femur or humerus.

The Association of Cancer Online Resources has a new Web site for patients that provides information on the treatment of cancer pain <www.cancer-pain.org>. The site lists medications, treatment options, and provides advice on how to communicate with physicians. It also has an interactive area where patients and caregivers can exchange knowledge with each other.

SUMMARY AND CONCLUSIONS

Osteoarthritis, fibromyalgia, headache, chronic back problems, and cancer are the primary causes of 90 percent of all chronic pain syndromes. Treatments for any of these conditions should begin with regular doses of medication, that are safe and cause few side effects (such as acetaminophen). Nondrug therapy should also be considered, such as physical and occupational therapy, exercise, and attention to diet and weight. If possible, treatments that prevent the onset of pain (as in migraine headache) should be fully utilized. In conditions such as cancer, regular doses of narcotic pain relievers should be prescribed in adequate amounts to relieve ongoing pain, and additional doses should be prescribed to relieve breakthrough pain. Effective therapies now exist for most chronic pain syndromes. The key is learning how to administer drug and nondrug therapies at the right time and in the right amount to relieve pain, maintain function, and maximize quality of life.

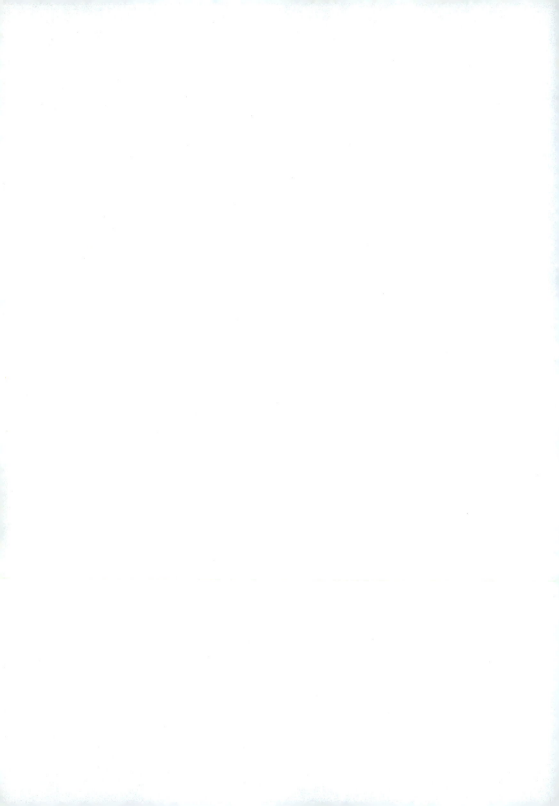

Chapter 14

Spiritual Approaches to Pain

This chapter focuses on spiritual beliefs, attitudes, and practices to help reduce the intensity of pain, improve coping, and stimulate psychological and spiritual growth. It is a personal account, written primarily for those who struggle with unrelieved chronic pain. Of all the things I've tried to cope with pain and disability, the spiritual approach by far has been the most helpful. I speak with authority in this chapter not because of any theological training (I have none), but because I am a practicing and committed Christian, because I have wrestled with pain and disability for many years, and because I have experience and training as a physician and as a counselor, working in the trenches with those who live with pain.

Spiritual strategies can provide a huge and often untapped source of comfort and relief for those experiencing chronic pain. Spiritual practices can change attitudes toward pain and thereby reduce suffering. The process, though, raises a number of difficult questions. How can unrelieved chronic pain possibly serve a spiritual purpose? Can pain be transformed into something that gives life meaning? How does a person with chronic pain pray and what might he or she pray for? What does it mean to be healed? These questions and more are addressed herein.

A SPIRITUAL ATTITUDE TOWARD PAIN

Chronic pain can be viewed as a huge unchangeable mountain. There is a way, however, to move the mountain, or at least to diminish its apparent size. The way to move the mountain is to change the way it is viewed. The mountain will become smaller or larger depending on how you perceive and understand it. The same applies to pain. Although you cannot decide whether to have pain, you can decide what your attitude toward it will be. A very real choice, then, confronts us. We must choose whether to view pain as a blessing or a curse. This choice must be made deliberately.

On one hand, we can choose to give in to the quite natural tendency to become frustrated, angry, and despondent; to withdraw from others into our own private world; and to view pain as an enemy that must be escaped from at any cost. This choice requires no effort, comes naturally, and usually leads to a downward spiral of worsening pain and depression, particularly if nothing can be done to safely relieve the pain. On the other hand, we can choose to develop a spiritual attitude toward pain. This latter choice does not come naturally. It takes considerable effort and discipline to avoid the all too natural slide toward seeing pain as an insurmountable, unmovable mountain.

What exactly is a spiritual attitude toward pain? I believe it has four components: submission, acceptance, understanding, and recognition of calling.

Submission

This is a difficult pill for most people to take, since human nature makes us intensely independent and self-serving, something our culture encourages and supports. By submission I mean exactly that: to stop everything for a moment and consciously decide to submit to God and to his plan for your life, whatever it may be and however much pain may be involved. It means to stop complaining about the pain, and stop blaming yourself, others, or God. This conscious decision to submit involves turning one's life over to God, fully embracing him, and pledging to spend the rest of one's life serving him. He says, "Take my yoke upon you and learn from me, for I am gentle and humble in heart, and you will find rest for your souls. For my yoke is easy and my burden is light" (Matthew 11:29-30). That burden, I guarantee, is a lot lighter than the one Mr. Pain wants to put on us. Submission is absolutely essential, and without it nothing in the rest of this chapter will make much sense. The decision to submit is not simply a one-time event but rather a continual, ongoing process of repeatedly submitting to God during the many moments of decision in the path of life ahead—especially during the difficult moments.

The power that is generated by submitting in this way is truly incredible, for with it comes a promise: "No test or temptation that comes your way is beyond the course of what others have had to face. All you need to remember is that God will never let you down; he'll never let you be pushed past your limits; he'll always be there to help you come through it" (1 Corinthians 10:13).[1] If you doubt this, read the fascinating book about Christian martyrs titled *Jesus Freaks*.[2] This book presents detailed accounts of the deaths of martyrs throughout the ages who, with lives submitted to God, were beaten, dismembered, burned, or otherwise tortured. Joy, peace, and God's presence were almost uniformly reported when pain was at its greatest. Somehow, the pain itself became transformed into these ecstatic human emotions. Submission of your life, your whole life, to God may transform your pain in the same way.

Being submitted to God also means relating to God on a more intimate level as master, counselor, and friend. This is a crucial step in developing a spiritual attitude toward pain. That relationship will sustain you during your darkest times, help to ease the frustration caused by unrelieved pain, bring back a sense of control, and diminish loneliness. It will direct and energize you. This relationship with the Divine is nourished by worship, study of Scripture, and prayer, and is the power source that will enable you to carry out the very difficult next steps that follow.

Acceptance

First, let me reaffirm my belief that every effort should be made to relieve pain, including getting the most comprehensive medical evaluation possible, using the latest proven pharmacological, surgical, psychological, social, and behavioral treatments available, and even trying some unproven alternative treatments. I have taken prescription medicine, switched medicines, consulted doctors, switched doctors, taken herbs, worn magnets, and paid attention to diet, weight, exercise, and sleep. I've reduced the stress in my life by trying to nourish family relationships and limit my job responsibilities. I've done everything possible to reduce my pain medically and to live a life that minimizes factors that might worsen the pain. Thus, I fully support and advise an exhaustive attempt to diagnose and alleviate pain, which includes praying that God will miraculously heal the cause of the pain and completely remove it.

There comes a time, however, when one must accept the pain and disability that remain, the pain that cannot be eradicated through sensible medical, psychological, surgical, and spiritual approaches. This means accepting the limitations that chronic pain has placed on life and deciding to live within those restrictions. Life has changed and may never be the same. Some activities that previously gave life meaning, purpose, joy, a sense of self-worth and dignity simply cannot be done anymore. Life has changed, and to dwell in the past is deadly.

Acceptance is different from resignation and giving up—very different. Acceptance involves a conscious choice to bear the cross that has been given—to bear it willingly and with head held high. It also never closes the door on the possibility or hope that God will someday relieve the pain either through his sovereign will or through some newly discovered drug or surgical treatment.

Acceptance involves turning pain that cannot be relieved over to God, and trusting that He will take care of it, not constantly worrying and obsessing over it. The kind of trust I'm talking about depends on a relationship with God. For example, if I have a colleague whom I know well and have learned I can count on, then I will be more confident to entrust him or her with an important responsibility. I will be less likely to worry about the situation since I know through past experience that he or she can be relied on. If I don't know the colleague or his or her abilities very well, I will be more likely to worry about what will happen, want to check on the situation myself, and if things aren't going immediately as planned, be tempted to take over the responsibility. Knowing God through a process of continually relating to Him in worship, Scripture, and prayer helps develop faith and confidence in His ability to take care of things.

This process of doing everything one can to treat the pain, and then accepting what remains and trusting God to take care of it, is a delicate one requiring wisdom and judgment. Knowing at what point we have done our part, knowing when we have done everything possible within our power to rectify the situation, and then letting go, is the challenge. This challenge is perhaps best summarized by Reinhold Niebuhr in the serenity prayer: "O God, grant me the serenity to accept the things I cannot change, the courage to change the things I can, and the wisdom to know the difference." We all need help "to know the difference."

Understanding

With acceptance of pain must come a certain understanding: within this new, seemingly more limited world one has decided to live in, every positive emotion ever experienced in the past is still possible. This fact, for some, may be a stunning realization. It means the greatest joys and feelings of happiness, the deepest sense of peace, the most stunning moments of wonder and awe ever experienced are still possible. It means the deepest sense of meaning and purpose and vision for a future is still possible. It means the closest and deepest personal relationships with others are still possible. It means the experience of God's presence and love, as real as ever before, is still possible. Many of these deeply positive and meaningful experiences may even be more possible now than in one's previous life because much of the old baggage is no longer a hindrance.

Chronic pain can help to redirect our focus to the things that really matter. It can motivate us to reach outward and inward toward sources of strength we wouldn't have turned to unless forced to. When we develop the right attitude, we sometimes discover ourselves finally arriving at a place we had been searching for in our old life without success. Chronic pain can make us more real, more sensitive, more humble, more fully human than ever before. This is the great potential of pain. Remember, though, that pain can also do the exact opposite, if allowed to take its natural course unopposed by the human will to embark on this more narrow, seemingly difficult higher path.

Calling

The final component of a spiritual attitude toward pain is to view the pain as a special calling. Yes, you read correctly: a *special calling*. That may seem ridiculous to some of us who see pain as an unwanted parasite sapping our strength. How can pain be a calling, let alone a special calling, one to be utilized for a higher purpose? The majority of people on this planet go through life without experiencing a great deal of physical pain. For some reason, though, God has allowed a number of us to experience chronic, disabling pain. Why? Or why me? This question is often asked by chronic pain sufferers.

I believe an answer is that we've been called to serve God in a specific way, one that only those who struggle with pain day after day have the ability to do. In fact, it is the very struggle with pain itself which equips us with the tools necessary to serve in this manner. Those tools can't be acquired except through the frustration and agony of the pain experience. Chronic pain provides unique insights and understanding that most people without pain don't have and can't relate to. This gives those who experience pain a unique ability to understand and speak to others who struggle with chronic pain. There are millions of such people out there who need understanding, compassion, kindness, support, encouragement, hope, and vision for what is possible, even if their pain never goes away. We are the ones who have been called to help meet those needs.

If we accept this calling, then every ache and every twinge of pain will serve to remind us of why we are here. Rather than drain life of its purpose, pain will instead help to infuse it with meaning. Rather than see pain as a punishment for past sins, mistakes, or errors, or as a random act by a cruel devil or god, it is possible to come to a place where we can see pain almost as a blessing. Coming to that place is not easy, and the stories told of those with chronic pain in previous chapters testify to the challenge. It is a process that involves a lot of conscious effort, discipline, faith, and trust—trust that we were not just created to endure lives of meaningless suffering.

Would it be all that unusual if that were the case? Have you ever had a particular trait you'd like to be rid of, but which turned out to be advantageous in the long run? We are all very different from one another. Each of us has different talents, abilities, and strengths. Similarly, each of us has unique vulnerabilities, weaknesses, and inadequacies. It is our talents and natural abilities that are usually seen as our greatest strengths. Attractive physical appearance, strength and balance, skill at conversation and speech, knowledge, shrewdness in business and management—these are things that often attract attention.

Many times, however, it is exactly these natural talents that end up being the greatest sources of sorrow. Also, seeming defects, weaknesses, and difficult life circumstances, which are pitied by the outside world, can be sources of strength and key to building character. This is possible, too, with chronic pain if we can view it with a spiritual attitude and use that pain to transform our lives.

The following story, "The Donkey," offers a positive message.[3]

> One day, a farmer's donkey fell down into a well. The animal cried pitifully for hours as the farmer tried to figure out what to do. Finally, he decided that the animal was old and the well needed to be covered up anyway, so it just wasn't worth it to retrieve the donkey.
>
> So he invited all his neighbors to come over and help him. They all grabbed a shovel and began to shovel dirt into the well. At first, the donkey realized what was happening and cried horribly. Then, to everyone's amazement, he quieted down. A few shovel loads later, the farmer finally looked down the well and was astonished at what he saw.
>
> With every shovel of dirt that hit his back, the donkey was doing something quite remarkable. He would shake it off and take a step up. As the farmer's neighbors continued to shovel dirt on top of the animal, he would shake it off and take a step up. Pretty soon, everyone was amazed as the donkey stepped up over the edge of the well and trotted off!

The moral of this story is that you can be sure that life is going to shovel dirt on you—all kinds of dirt. The trick to getting out of the well is to shake it off and take a step up. Each of our troubles is a stepping-stone. We can get out of the deepest well just by not stopping, by never giving up—by using pain itself to help us develop a spiritual attitude not only to pain alone but to every other adversity we face in life.

Edith Schaefer wrote a marvelous book in 1978 with the simple title *Affliction*.[4] In that book she describes how tremendous victory can be accomplished in the midst of unchanging circumstances, how God and his legions of angels, the great saints and martyrs, and millions of others who have passed on before us (including deceased loved ones) are watching anxiously how we respond to the challenges presented to us. Will we curse God or praise Him in our circumstances? The crowd roars with approval when we carry our pain with dignity and refuse to be tempted into discouragement, complaining, or resentment. Each time we praise God, each time we submit to His will for our lives, each time we reach out in kindness to others in pain—the victory banner raises in heaven and all rejoice. That victory is in every way equivalent to the victory that occurs when God miraculously takes away a person's pain. Because the battle is often a harder one, the rejoicing is even louder and more exuberant. The opportunity for victory in the spiritual realm, then, may be greater during unrelieved pain than at any other time in life. It is up to us to either take up the call to arms or retreat in defeat.

Three spiritual activities help both to reinforce a spiritual attitude and to bring about either a lessening of pain or a lessening of the suffering that accompanies pain. These activities are participation and worship in a faith community, study of Scripture, and conversing with God in prayer.

FAITH COMMUNITY INVOLVEMENT

Chronic pain in a person's life naturally tends to focus attention away from what is going on in the lives of others. Furthermore, pain-induced disability and mobility restrictions tend to limit social interactions. It is more difficult to go places, attend meetings, and participate in recreational activities through which social relationships form and are maintained. If a person is also struggling with depression, poor self-esteem, and a sense of despair over seemingly unending misery, the desire to socialize will rapidly diminish. All of these factors contribute to a tendency toward social withdrawal. This tendency to withdraw from others into the self must be carefully monitored and consciously resisted.

Participation and worship in a religious community is necessary because of a universal human need to interact with other people, which cannot go unfulfilled without consequences. English poet John Donne summarized it succinctly when he wrote, "No man is an island, entire of itself." Like it or not, we are all connected. What we do affects others for good or for bad, just as what others do affects us. There is actually biological evidence that proves separating ourselves from others has negative consequences. Many studies in both humans and primates show that social isolation causes changes in the immune system, endocrine system, and cardiovascular system—the very processes in the body that protect us from disease and help our bodies re-cover from illness.[5] In addition, social isolation results in altered thinking and mental aberrations that have negative effects on emotions and perceptions.

Participation in the faith community is also important because it is emphasized in Scripture. Consider the entire nation of Israel meeting regularly at the tabernacle to sacrifice, or Jesus meeting with his disciples to teach and fellowship with them, or the early Christians meeting regularly to eat together and worship. The apostle Paul said it plainly, "Let us not give up meeting together, as some are in the habit of doing, but let us encourage one another" (Hebrews 10:25). Why is this so? Because we physically, mentally, and spiritually need fellowship, support, and encouragement from our community of faith. Perhaps even more important, the community of faith *needs us*.

Needs us? Needs people with chronic pain and disability? Yes, they need us. Not only do they need us present so they can minister to us (how else can a people of faith carry out their ministry of "Love thy neighbor" if there is no neighbor to love?), they also need us to minister *to them*. As we learn to successfully bear the burden of chronic pain, we need to act as both comforters and witnesses to others in the faith community who are themselves coping with unique troubles in life. Although they may not be dealing with chronic physical pain, I guarantee you that most are dealing with some kind of difficult situation, worry, or problem. They, too, need our support, encouragement, and listening ear. For our own mental, physical, and spiritual health, we need to be there to provide it.

Power for strength and healing is generated when the faith community comes together to worship. Scripture repeatedly confirms this: "For where two or three come together in my name, there am I with them" (Matthew 18:20). Although God is always with us, whether alone or with others, Jesus believed that it was important enough to point out to His disciples that there was something special about coming together as a group to worship and pray. Likewise, consider the instruction in the book of James: "Is any one of you sick? He should call the elders of the church to pray over him and anoint him with oil in the name of the Lord. And the prayer offered in faith will make the sick person well; the Lord will raise him up. If he has sinned, he will be forgiven. Therefore confess your sins to each other and pray for each other so that you may be healed" (James 5:14-16). It can't be any clearer than that. Those of us in pain need to confess to one another, pray for one another, and support one another.

SCRIPTURE

The Holy Scriptures are an unparalleled source of direction, comfort, and hope for those with chronic pain. A huge part of the Bible is about people suffering and overcoming adversity. Consider Abraham and Sarah's struggle to have a child, Isaac, and then the threatened loss of that child when being asked by God to sacrifice him. Consider Jacob and the suffering he endured when he thought his favored son Joseph had been devoured by a wild animal. Consider Joseph being thrown in prison for resisting temptation and doing the right thing. Consider the entire nation of Israel in bondage to slavery in Egypt for centuries. Consider the wanderings of the Jewish nation for forty years in the desert, and later the destruction of Jerusalem and exile of its inhabitants to a foreign land. Consider the physical pain and suffering Jesus endured on the cross, the stoning of Stephen by the angry crowd, and Paul and Peter imprisoned in Rome, to name just a few examples. In fact, the entire book of Job is devoted to suffering, both physical and psychological, and the Book of Psalms deals much with sorrow and depression. Here are role models of people who continued on despite their pain, many eventually triumphing as they lived their lives according to a certain set of principles that God revealed to them. These principles are timeless keys to human fulfillment and happiness in all situations, but especially when the going gets rough.

In addition to containing role models for triumphing over adversity, I believe Scripture also contain words that produce healing. At least sixty separate Scriptures speak of healing, health, and wholeness (see Appendix I). Rather than filling our minds with doubts, complaints, memories of the way it used to be, or envy of those who are healthy and without pain, it would be better to fill our thoughts with healing Scriptures that provide the promises of God to those who believe. Indeed, "For as he thinks in his heart, so is he" (Proverbs 23:7 [KJV]).

One of the most common forms of secular psychotherapy today for the treatment of depression and anxiety is cognitive therapy. Cognitive therapy seeks to replace ruminative, exaggerated, negative, pessimistic thinking with positive, wholesome, truthful thoughts. This is not a new idea. The Scriptures repeatedly emphasize the need for this. Jesus said, "For out of the heart [mind] come evil thoughts, murder, adultery, sexual immorality, theft, false testimony, slander. These are what make a man 'unclean'" (Matthew 15:19). The apostle Paul said, "Finally, brothers, whatever is true, whatever is noble, whatever is right, whatever is pure, whatever is lovely, whatever is admirable—if anything is excellent or praiseworthy—think about such things" (Philippians 4:8). Certainly, the Scriptures are true, right, pure, and lovely, are they not? Let us fill our minds with the healing words of Scripture, not the lies of inadequacy and helplessness.

PRAYER

Prayer is the most important weapon we have against pain. It is easy, however, to underestimate its power. Prayer doesn't cost anything, is always available, and doesn't require much training or skill. Even little children can pray. Because it is so easy and readily accessible, we often take it for granted and fail to recognize what an amazing privilege it is and what truly incredible things it can do. Perhaps the most important thing it can do is to bring us closer to God. It is within that relationship that the power lies.

What to Pray For

What should people with chronic pain pray for? Depending on one's theology, some might be reluctant to pray for relief of pain. They may see pain as God's will for them. Others may see pain as just punishment for sins committed in the past. Still others may believe that God doesn't intervene in the world, and that it is not respectful to ask God for things such as simple earthly comfort. These people may pray for God's will in their situation, and for strength to bear the cross that has been given them. They do not expect to be healed and do not request it. I imagine, though, that most people pray for pain relief and for physical healing—often out of desperation, as I have done so often. It is difficult to know, then, what to pray for. Here are some suggestions.

Pray for the Strength to Make God First

Traditional Jews, Christians, and Muslims would all agree to this. The first of the Ten Commandments requires it: "I am the Lord thy God, which have brought thee out of the land of Egypt, out of the house of bondage. Thou shalt have no other gods before me" (Exodus 20:2-3 [KJV]). Jesus emphasized it in the New Testament as the most important of all the commandments ("'Love the Lord your God with all your heart and with all your soul and with all your mind.' This is the first and greatest commandment"—Matthew 22:37-38). Nothing, then, should become more important, more central, more consuming of your time and attention than God. Recall that this is also the first step in developing a spiritual attitude.

If we allow anything else to become central and ultimate, our lives will quickly become unbalanced. If that has occurred, then we must confess it, receive forgiveness, and put God back into the place He belongs, putting everything else after and below Him—*including pain*. Pray that God will give everything you need to put Him first. Having that balance of priorities will provide an emotional stability and power otherwise not possible.

Even if God doesn't relieve the pain, be assured that He will listen, understand, and give us sufficient strength to bear it. Jesus experienced such pain that He sweat drops of blood, and was physically tortured to the point of exhaustion and ultimately death. As a man, He felt deserted and alone at the moment of His greatest agony: "And about the ninth hour Jesus cried with a loud voice, saying, 'Eli, Eli, lama sabachthani?' that is to say, My God, my God, why hast thou forsaken me?" (Matthew 27:46 [KJV]). Sound familiar? Yes, He knows what pain and suffering are like. Isaiah 53:3 says, "He is despised and rejected of men; a man of sorrows, and acquainted with grief . . . he was despised, and we esteemed him not."

He knows what not being understood is like too. Even His closest friends and companions, His disciples, did not really understand why He had come, despite all the teaching and time He spent with them. They thought that He would free them of Roman rule, that His kingdom would be of this world. His closest friend, Peter, wanted to stop Him from carrying out the very task for which He had come. No one really understood Him during his life as a man. Yes, He knows what it's like not to be understood.

Just as Jesus was given sufficient strength and help to bear His cross, so also God has promised this for us. After three times refusing to take the apostle Paul's "thorn in my flesh" away, God said to Him "My grace is sufficient" (2 Corinthians 12:7,9). God gives us the strength and grace sufficient to bear the burden of pain. When God is first in our lives, it is to him that we go to meet that need. Do you expect friends and family to provide you with the comfort and understanding you need to deal with your pain? If so, you've probably already discovered that such expectations are seldom realized. If you expect those who have not experienced physical pain to show compassion, especially over the long term, you will be disappointed. If you have frustrations or struggles, share them with God first—He is the one who really knows and understands your situation and is able to do something about it. Go to God first for every need you have, and then give to others of what you get there.

Pray for a Closer Walk

By asking God for things that we need—including relief of physical pain and emotional suffering—we acknowledge our dependence on Him for all things. Because He loves us, though, He may not always give us what we want. Rather, He gives us what we *need*. What do we really need? If God really exists and has a special plan for each of our lives, what is our greatest need? Is it not to walk close to God so that we will know and have the power to carry out His special plan for our lives? Is a full, satisfying, and meaningful experience here on earth possible without that? With God by our side, I believe a full life is possible even if it includes a life with pain (recall Jackie's comments in Chapter 6). Let us pray, then, for whatever we need to come closer to Him. Sometimes pain is necessary for that to occur. No doubt it is difficult to realize, especially when we are in pain, that anything good could possibly come out of it.

I have a five-year-old daughter, Rebekah. I love her as much as anything I can imagine. The other day she got a wooden splinter in her finger when she was playing out on the deck. She showed it to me, and I realized it had to come out. If it didn't come out, the finger would probably get infected, cause even greater pain in the days ahead, and possibly lead to worse problems. However, she didn't want to go through the pain necessary for the splinter to come out. She didn't understand the good that would result from the pain necessary to get the splinter out. She didn't want me to take that splinter out, and I didn't want to take it out and cause her all that pain. But because of my love for her, because I knew that the best thing for her was to get the splinter out, I had to do it—as painful as it was for both of us. Are things really all that different with God? The splinter is our selfishness, pride, and desire to go our own way. It's a splinter that needs to come out, a splinter that will separate us from God and ultimately destroy us.

Sometimes, though, pain seems to last for seemingly no good reason. Why does God allow this? This reminds me of an anonymous story recently sent to me.[6]

> A man was sleeping at night in his cabin when suddenly his room filled with light, and God appeared. God told the man He had work for him to do, and showed him a large rock in front of his cabin. God explained that the man was to push against the rock with all his might. So, this the man did, day after day. For many years he toiled from sunup to sundown; his shoulders set squarely against the cold, massive surface of the unmoving rock, pushing with all of his might.
>
> Each night the man returned to his cabin sore and worn out, feeling that his whole day had been spent in vain. Since the man was getting discouraged, self-doubt and defeatism entered the picture by placing thoughts into his weary mind: "You have been pushing against that rock for a long time, and it hasn't moved." These thoughts gave the man the impression that the task was impossible and that he was a failure. These thoughts discouraged and disheartened the man. "Why kill myself over this?" he thought. "I'll put in my time, giving just the minimum effort; and that will be good enough." And that is what he planned to do, until one day he decided to make it a matter of prayer and take his troubled thoughts to God.
>
> "Dear God" he said, "I have labored long and hard in Your service, putting all my strength to do that which You have asked.

Yet, after all this time, I have not even budged that rock by half a millimeter. What is wrong? Why am I failing?"

The Lord responded compassionately, "My child, when I asked you to serve Me and you accepted, I told you that your task was to push against the rock with all of your strength, which you have done. Never once did I mention to you that I expected you to move it. Your task was to push.

"And now you come to Me with your strength spent, thinking that you have failed, but is that really so? Look at yourself. Your arms are strong and muscled, your back sinewy and brown, your hands are callused from constant pressure, your legs have become massive and hard. Through opposition you have grown much, and your abilities now surpass that which you used to have. Yet you haven't moved the rock. But your calling was to be obedient and to push and to exercise your faith and trust in My wisdom. This you have done. Now I, My child, will now move the rock."

Pain, then, can be used as an instrument to make us stronger and move us closer to God so that we will become more compassionate, more merciful, more understanding. It may seem as though nothing is being accomplished, but if we bear the burden of pain willingly and patiently as we seek to come closer to Him, God can use it for our greatest good.

Pray for Faith

Sometimes God does relieve our pain in a mysterious and miraculous way according to His will, defying all logic and understanding. Most of the time He does so in response to prayer and uses our faith to accomplish this. Scientists are now just discovering the power of belief and what strong expectations of healing can accomplish. Indeed, we may be "wired for God."[7] From earlier chapters, we know there are direct connections between the brain (the center of our faith and will) and the places in the spinal cord ("gates") that pain transmissions must pass through to reach our consciousness. Thus there is every reason to believe that strong faith in God's ability to relieve pain could unconsciously send impulses from the brain down to the spinal cord and other pain-sensing areas to limit or stop the transmission of pain. In this way, pain could be either lessened or blocked completely.

The brain is also connected by the nervous system to every organ and limb in the body, including the immune system and the cardiovascular system. Thus, direct physiological connections exist by which our minds can directly impact the body's functions, including the natural systems that speed healing. Faith in God's power and ability to heal may activate those very systems that were designed by Him to accomplish self-repair and healing. In this way, the diseases responsible for chronic pain could also be favorably influenced.

Physiological pathways exist in the body by which faith and trust in God can ignite real changes that result in pain relief and physical healing. I see no reason why God would not use the marvelous bodies He has created to heal us, nor any reason not to pray for such healing. But sometimes God does not respond to our persistent pleas for pain relief, regardless of how much we pray or how much faith we have. What then?

Pray for Wholeness

It is important to understand what it really means when we ask God to heal us. Otherwise, when we pray for healing, how will we know when we receive it? Many restrict their definition of healing to *physical* healing: the unexplained recovery from a life-threatening disease, the miraculous cure of cancer, and, for us in particular, the sudden disappearance of long-standing pain. This, they say, is the only true sign of victory, of triumph of God over evil and disease. Healing does include miraculous physical cures, but it also involves much more than that. In fact, physical healing may be relatively low on God's priority list of things that need healing in our lives.

Remember that God stands outside of time, which enables Him to see into the past from the beginning of time and into the future to the end of time. The short seventy or eighty years of life that we spend on earth likely represents only an infinitesimal fraction of the eternity in which our souls will find themselves after our human existence ends. Certainly no one knows for sure what happens after death, but most major religions in the world believe there is *something*. Almost without exception, those same religions teach that whatever we accomplish here on earth affects our conditions then. Indeed, some of the most important accomplishments may have very little to do with our physical comfort.

Indeed, everyone is destined to die—even those who experience miraculous healings. Perhaps they are spared a few years, but they will all eventually die. From God's perspective, then, other things may be much more important than either our physical health or our freedom from pain. In fact, it is quite likely that only when our physical health is threatened do we pay attention to those things of greatest value: the kind of lifestyle we are living, our relationships with family and friends, our concern and compassion for others, our relationship with God. Adversity, then, may redirect our attention to those things truly and eternally significant.

When we pray for healing, God may decide to heal us in other areas of our lives. He may enable us to confess and receive forgiveness for past errors and mistakes. He may enable us to forgive and release others who have hurt us, whom we have resented and held hostage by our grudges. He may enable us for the first time to experience compassion for others in pain, and arouse in us a desire to help and understand them. He may answer our prayer for healing by allowing us to experience His presence in the midst of our pain, as He did with Job during his trials. He may answer our prayers by allowing us to discover a spiritual world that we never thought existed, nor would have looked for, unless our physical circumstances had forced us to open our eyes.

Healing means "to make whole." There are millions of people who walk this earth completely without pain and yet are not whole. Their lives are fractured by unforgiveness, resentment, greed, selfishness, anger, anxiety, depression, hopelessness, and lack of purpose. Many perfectly healthy people without any physical pain kill themselves every year because their lives are so disordered they choose to end them rather than to continue to live on. Indeed, let us pray for healing, for wholeness, and pray for it from God's perspective, not our own.

Pray for the Ability to Love

In addition to making God first, walking closer to him, having more faith, and seeking real healing and wholeness, let us pray for the ability to love others by showing greater kindness and more understanding toward them. Chronic pain often makes people irritable, cranky, and anything but loving and kind toward others. The burden of pain frequently makes us touchy, reduces our flexibility, and shrinks our ability to tolerate others, especially their quirks and differences. It makes us hypersensitive to others when they fail us or show lack of understanding. Pain and disability, however, cannot excuse us from loving others. Pray for the strength and the will to love others despite our natural feelings.

Corinthians 13 talks about love, and makes a huge point that is often not fully appreciated. The point is this: No matter how much knowledge, insight, and understanding we learn from our pain, without love all of it is worth nothing. No matter how much we suffer or endure, if we do not show love for others, it is a complete waste. Don't let your pain go to waste—pray for the strength to love and serve others God's way.

There are basically three kinds of love: filial love, eros love, and agape love. Filial love is the "if" kind of love: if you are nice to me, if you do things for me, if you make me feel good, then I will love you. Eros love is the "because" kind of love: I love you because you are beautiful, because you love me, because you are wealthy, famous, or respected. Agape love is the "in spite of" kind of love: I love you in spite of the fact that you can do nothing for me, that you are ungrateful, that you are irritating, that you are undependable, that you are untrustworthy.

The agape kind of love is what Corinthians 13:4-7 is talking about: "Love is patient, love is kind. It does not envy, it does not boast, it is not proud. It is not rude, it is not self-seeking, it is not easily angered, it keeps no record of wrongs. Love does not delight in evil but rejoices with the truth. It always protects, always trusts, always hopes, always perseveres." The agape kind of love is what Romans 13:10 is talking about: "Therefore love is the fulfillment of the law" (in other words, if you love others, you will find yourself automatically doing all that God expects of you). This is the kind of love that we are all supposed to show others—and no amount of chronic pain or suffering can excuse us from doing it. If we do not love others, we will reap negative consequences.

It is important for those of us in pain, again through an act of will, to decide to love others—even when we don't feel like it (which is most of the time at first). If we allow pain to prevent us from doing this, we will miss out on the many benefits and joys. Even more important, loving others around us (whoever they may be) in this unconditional way is the most powerful and effective weapon that can be used against chronic pain. I am convinced that much of the suffering that accompanies pain results from the natural (perhaps even biological) inclination to withdraw inward and focus attention on our pain rather than on the needs of others. Because we have such a great spiritual responsibility and human need to love others, whenever this stops (no matter what the reason), a deep void opens up in our lives and despair sets in. Don't allow pain to do this. Pray for the ability to love and be kind to others in the agape way.

Remember the story about Mr. Pain I told in Chapter 2? How did the fellow Anyone find relief in the giant's prison? It was by reaching out to the person beside him who was in pain. By comforting his neighbor, Anyone was himself comforted.

How I Pray

Most will agree there is no special formula or prayer technique that always ensures results. There are, however, a few basic underlying principles. Time must be set aside to pray alone on a regular basis. The environment one chooses to pray in should be quiet. The physical position one takes when praying should be relaxed but not conducive to sleep. Pray when alert, not sleepy or tired. Praying sincerely from the heart is perhaps most basic and necessary. Other than that, each person should develop a way of praying that fits his or her unique personality and situation. I describe next how I pray and what prayer means to me. This is the right way of praying for me, and perhaps only me. But at least it will provide an example of how one person familiar with chronic pain prays.

For me, prayer is a simple conversation. It is a time I set aside to meet with God and communicate with Him. I talk, He listens; He talks, I listen. It's a two-way street, similar to any other conversation with a close friend.

First, I talk. Prayer for me begins with adoration and worship. I recognize who God is—the Creator of everything that has ever been and that will ever be; the Person who first thought of me and brought me into being; the One whom I will leap toward at the moment when my death arrives and whose strong and loving arms will catch me. This is the God who deserves my worship, not my job, my possessions, my obsessive wants and needs, nor my pain. It is amazing indeed that He who is far greater than all the world's presidents, emperors, and leaders wants to meet with me and be a part of my life. And oh, how I need Him. Only He can give me the strength to keep fighting, keep enduring, keep loving, keep hoping.

Next, I recognize who I am, which involves confession. I confess all of the selfish decisions, thoughts, and strivings that have hurt others. I confess pride, arrogance, and lack of kindness and compassion. I confess worry over things that really don't matter. I confess my lack of attention to God during the day. I confess that I have allowed pain to have the upper hand in my life, that I have not trusted enough nor been faithful enough in bearing the cross that I have been given. I confess that I have complained, questioned, and demanded to be released from my burden of pain. I acknowledge that I am continually missing the target God has set before me—that of a fulfilling, victorious, abundant life of service to Him and to others. I admit that I am constantly straying off the path to abundant life. I need confession, for this helps me to recognize that I have indeed wandered and gives me the resolve to get back on the path—free of guilt and energized to start anew.

Then I express thanks. Yes, there are so many things to be thankful for! I have been blessed indeed—with physical health (yes, physical health), with mental health, with a comfortable house to live in, plenty of food, a devoted wife and two beautiful children, other caring family members, friends and colleagues, a fulfilling job, living free in the greatest nation in the world, and more than anything else, faith in and a relationship with the Divine who gives my life purpose and direction. I am so thankful. I'm also thankful for the pain and limitations, for the trials and difficulties each day that help to mold me into the kind of person that God wants me to become—so much to be thankful for, so very much.

Finally, I ask God for help. I ask God to protect my wife and children from physical or emotional harm, and to walk closely alongside them during the day and throughout the night. I ask for spiritual, physical, and emotional health for my mother, who must care for my ailing father, completely immobilized by a massive stroke, and especially for my father, locked in his body, unable to speak or even to swallow. I ask for blessings for my friends and co-workers, and for the many whom I have promised I would pray. I ask for health, strength, and healing in my own physical body, so that I might be free of pain and limitation. I ask for wisdom and insight to solve the problems I must face that day, and for kindness in everything I do. I ask for greater faith and trust, so that I will not worry about the present or the future. If physical healing is God's will for me, I ask that my lack of faith may not hinder it. I pray for strength to make God first in my life and to love others as He does. There is so much that I need from my Father.

I conclude my part of the conversation in prayer with a final request, that God would bless me. I ask to be blessed with everything that has been planned for me since the very moment that my Creator made me: blessed with an abundant life filled with purpose and meaning and love. Is that possible for someone in chronic pain? Jesus has already responded to that question: "With man this is impossible, but with God all things are possible" (Matthew 19:26). Even when pain is screaming for attention, even when pain is threatening to overwhelm and suffocate me—even then, I know that the abundant life is possible if I keep my inner eye focused on Him.

Then I listen. It's God's turn to talk. As a five-year-old boy secretly confided to his grandfather one day, "You know, Grandpa, when I go to bed at night it gets really dark and really quiet in my room. If I hold my breath, lay very still, and listen, I hear Jesus talking." The little boy could hear Jesus talking. That small quiet voice in the night. What a beautiful illustration describing the time to be quiet and silent in prayer, to listen for God's voice.

During this time of meditation, I try hard to clear my mind of extraneous thoughts and worries. This is difficult for me because precisely at that time it seems as though a flood of thoughts gush in. It helps to have some kind of object on which to focus my attention. I sometimes use a crucifix or an image of Jesus kneeling in the garden of Gethsemane. At other times I will pick out a verse in the Bible and meditate on that, allowing God to speak to me through the Scripture (many of the Scriptures in Appendix I have helped me this way). God may also respond to me at other times during the day, through my own thoughts, as I confront challenging circumstances or difficult decisions.

Scientific research actually shows that focused meditation ("Be still and know that I am God"—Psalm 46:10) can help to significantly reduce pain symptoms, alleviate depressed mood, and improve other psychological symptoms.[9] In that study, pain-related drug use decreased and self-esteem increased. The improvement occurred in both men and women and in those with different kinds of pain. Although meditation is often thought of as a Hindu, Buddhist, or New Age practice, this spiritual activity actually has a rather long and deep tradition within the Christian church.[10]

For me, prayer is spending time with the closest friend I will ever have in this life or the next. I wouldn't have recognized my need for such a friend if it weren't for my pain, which forced me to seek Him because I was desperate and had nowhere else to turn. He has been a true friend, one that has helped dispel loneliness, fear, and isolation during my darkest hours.

Praying in Severe Pain

When pain is severe, prayer need not be elaborate or prolonged. Sometimes, a simple "Help me, Lord" is all that can be uttered. These prayers are heard, too—and they are enough. At such times of severe pain, however, the faith of even the most devout person is likely to be tested. In fact, God may seem strangely absent or nonresponsive to desperate pleas for relief by us and by our loved ones. Sometimes we are forced to fly awhile on our own to strengthen our wings of faith. It is often not until afterward, when looking back at the entire situation, that we realize God was indeed there and very close. We simply couldn't "feel" His presence or perhaps recognize Him. Sometimes He comes in the form of a family member, friend, or even a religious or health professional to stand close to us during those difficult times. Remember, though, God never leaves or abandons us—that He has promised.

SUMMARY AND CONCLUSIONS

Spiritual approaches to chronic pain are powerful and effective ways of both relieving pain and relieving the suffering that accompanies pain. Consciously cultivating a spiritual attitude toward pain is of primary importance, and is based upon submission, acceptance, understanding, and developing a sense of calling. Spiritual practices such as involvement in a faith community, studying Scripture, and conversing with God in prayer will not only help to develop and maintain a spiritual attitude but will also ignite spiritual and psychological growth. Then, whether the severity of the pain changes or not, at least you will change for the better.

What is the real reason we are here? Why have we been born at this time and period in history? Is it simply to live a long, healthy, fun-filled and easy life, free of pain, suffering, trials, and adversity? Is that why we are here? Once that is done for a few decades, should we simply die and pass away into nonexistence? Is that all there is? I don't believe so. I believe our primary goal in this life is to come to know, love, and serve God, to become more Christlike in character, and to love one another more completely and unconditionally. Chronic pain may help us to accomplish these goals—and if we can use it for that purpose then this truth more than any other will set us free from the prison of pain.

Chapter 15

Ten Practical Steps
for Slaying the Giant

According to experts in chronic pain, 90 percent of people can experience significant improvement in the control of their pain by following a relatively simple set of recommendations. That figure does not include additional gains possible by taking advantage of spiritual resources. This chapter describes ten practical steps for managing nonmalignant chronic pain (see Chapter 13 for management of cancer pain). The steps are listed in the order to be taken, and then discussed in detail. The steps are cumulative (e.g., each step assumes the implementation of all prior steps). If pain relief is achieved at any particular step, no further steps are necessary. The ten practical steps for managing nonmalignant pain are:

1. Obtain a comprehensive medical evaluation
2. Use simple, safe drugs and noninvasive treatments
3. Exercise and pay attention to diet and weight
4. Consider inexpensive and safe alternative therapies
5. Try nonsteroidal anti-inflammatory drugs (NSAIDs)
6. Consider psychotherapy and behavioral treatments
7. Add low-dose antidepressants, gabapentin, or muscle relaxants
8. Seek treatment in a chronic pain clinic
9. Consider surgical therapies or other mechanical treatments
10. Consider narcotic analgesics

STEP 1: COMPREHENSIVE MEDICAL EVALUATION

Any type of pain, particularly if it is prolonged, requires a comprehensive medical evaluation. This often includes a careful neurological or other medical specialty evaluation to determine the exact cause of the pain. Once the cause is identified, a surgical evaluation may be needed to determine whether a simple surgical procedure may relieve the problem. Many people with years of chronic pain may never have had such a comprehensive evaluation. If such an evaluation has not been done, then a chronic pain specialist should be consulted to complete the kind of assessment described in Chapter 8. The choice of treatment for pain is highly dependent on the exact nature and cause of the pain, which makes it essential to have the correct diagnosis. Sometimes a second opinion is necessary, or even a third opinion, from a chronic pain expert located at a major medical center who will have the latest knowledge about the causes and treatments for pain. The American Pain Society has a Web site <http://www.ampainsoc. org/facility/> titled "Find a Pain Treatment Center" that can help identify locations of pain experts.

STEP 2: SIMPLE, SAFE DRUGS AND NONINVASIVE TREATMENTS

For persistent pain of any type, the medical treatment of first choice involves taking acetaminophen (Tylenol) for pain relief. This is the simplest and least toxic of all pain medications. Most people tolerate acetaminophen at doses up to 4,000 mg per day (two Extra-Strength Tylenol every six hours) without adverse side effects. This drug does not interact with other medications; does not cause constipation, nausea, or gastrointestinal irritation; and does not interfere with alertness or driving. Some people, however, are either allergic to acetaminophen (in rare cases) or have other medical problems involving the liver or kidney, which contraindicate its use. For chronic pain, acetaminophen should be taken on a regular schedule, not on an as-needed basis. Even simple over-the-counter drug therapies such as acetaminophen should be administered under the direction of a physician. Also, remember that over-the-counter preparations that contain aspirin are not recommended until Step 5, which is discussed later.

Application of heat and cold is simple and safe if used correctly. Applying an ice pack to an inflamed joint or a heating pad to a painful back will often bring considerable relief. Excessive use of heat or cold, however, can injure the skin and result in future problems. It is best to apply such treatments using some kind of protective layer on the skin and only for about twenty to thirty minutes at a time. Any prolonged redness of the skin after exposure indicates excessive use.

Transcutaneous electronic nerve stimulation (TENS) is noninvasive, has few if any side effects, and should be tried early on to see if any benefit results. TENS may also be considered after surgical procedures to help boost pain relief. This is particularly true for chronic low back pain.

STEP 3: EXERCISE AND ATTENTION TO DIET AND WEIGHT

Careful aerobic and stretching exercises, preferably based on a plan developed by a physical therapist, will help to maintain muscle flexibility, strength, and coordination. It will help to ensure bone strength and reduce the likelihood of developing osteoporosis. Regular exercise will help to keep weight down, thereby helping to relieve stress on painful joints or limbs, and will help to maintain cardiovascular tone. Finally, exercise will help to reduce psychological stress and improve self-image. Remember, however, that activity must be balanced with rest, and that some chronic pain conditions (such as inflammatory arthritis) may be made worse by prolonged, repetitive movements. Recommended exercise duration is twenty to thirty minutes three to five times per week. The exercise should be vigorous enough to increase the heart rate and respiratory rate. Some of the best kinds of exercise are swimming or aerobics in a heated pool, bicycle riding, and walking (if lower joints can handle the impact).

Regular times for sleep and relaxation should be included as part of the daily routine, including going to bed at the same time every night and getting up at the same time every morning. A twenty-minute nap in the afternoon after lunch may be beneficial (but before 2:00 p.m. and not for more than thirty minutes). Adaptive devices at work and around the house may take the stress and workload off painful joints. For example, those with painful wrists and fingers due to arthritis should consider obtaining voice-activated computer software that transfers the spoken word onto the screen (I use Dragon Naturally Speaking Preferred as my voice program, which allows me to create documents in Microsoft Word at about sixty words per minute with minimal use of my fingers or wrists). Be creative and find ways to increase functioning.

Attention to diet is also important to ensure adequate nutrition and to avoid excessive calorie intake. Raw fruits such as apples and oranges provide natural sugar for energy, vitamin C, and dietary fiber. Green leafy vegetables provide complex carbohydrates, minerals, dietary fiber, and are low in calories. White meat (turkey or chicken) and fish provide protein, essential minerals and vitamins, and are low in fat, providing good low-calorie nutrition. Cheese and milk products are good sources of protein and calcium, but are relatively high in calories and cholesterol, low in fiber, and may be constipating. White breads, starches, chips, and concentrated sweets are high in calories, low in dietary fiber, and low in vitamins and minerals, so they should be eaten sparingly. High intake of low-calorie fluids such as water or non-sweetened lemonade is encouraged to prevent the development of kidney stones and bladder infections. Avoid snacks between meals and especially at night before bed.

The goal is to eat a balanced diet distributed throughout the day in three or four small meals that are high in fluids, protein, complex carbohydrates, minerals, vitamins, dietary fiber (particularly if medications are being taken that cause constipation), and low in calories. These recommendations assume no other significant medical problems require the restriction of fluids, protein, or fiber.

STEP 4: INEXPENSIVE SAFE ALTERNATIVE THERAPIES

Choose an herbal preparation such as glucosamine or an omega-3 fatty acid supplement and take it at a sufficient dose for three months to see if it makes a difference. Be sure that the preparation you take actually has the right amount of active ingredient in it. If after three months a clear difference is not evident, stop it and try something else. Be sure that alternative medicines do not have adverse side effects that are not well known. This is particularly true if other medications are being taken that may interact with them.

Consider an alternative therapy such as acupuncture, massage, or even hypnosis, and again take the treatment for two or three months. Keep track of how much money is spent on these treatments, since costs can add up quickly, particularly if treatments are given more than once a week. Also, be clear about what you want from the therapist. If you simply want someone to listen to you and be kind, then try to meet these needs elsewhere at lower expense. Remember that the success of many of these treatments is because the therapist offers time and attention that patients have trouble getting from their health care professionals.

STEP 5: NONSTEROIDAL ANTI-INFLAMMATORY DRUGS (NSAIDs)

Step 5 is really the first stage at which treatments for chronic pain can begin to have serious side effects, so movement to this step should not occur until Steps 1 through 4 have been exhausted. Furthermore, some amount of physical pain may need to be accepted, particularly if the intensity is only mild and not significantly interfering with function. A decision to take NSAIDs over the long term should not be made before carefully considering other options, including no further treatment.

People with a history of stomach problems, ulcers, kidney or liver disease, or bleeding disorders should stay away from NSAIDs. If these health conditions are not present and a chronic pain condition exists in which inflammation plays a role (arthritis, fibromyalgia, back, and other musculoskeletal pain syndromes), then consider taking a NSAID. Because of fewer side effects and greater effectiveness in relieving pain, a COX-2 inhibitor (celecoxib, rofecoxib, or meloxicam) should be the first choice. Compared to the more traditional NSAIDs such as aspirin, ibuprofen, or naproxen, however, COX-2 inhibitors are more expensive, there is less long-term experience with these drugs, and people with sulfa allergy cannot take celecoxib (Celebrex).

Be aware that there is great individual variability in both pain response and tolerability to NSAIDs. For example, one person may tolerate ibuprofen quite well and receive good pain relief, whereas ibuprofen may not work for another person, who may receive great benefit from rofecoxib (Vioxx). Therefore, an NSAID should be taken for three or four weeks and then its effectiveness evaluated. If it doesn't work or side effects emerge, that one should be stopped and another NSAID tried. It is always best to start low and gradually increase the dose every few days to minimize side effects.

STEP 6: PSYCHOTHERAPY AND BEHAVIORAL TREATMENTS

If stress is playing a role, either causing or resulting from chronic pain, then Step 6 may need to come before Step 5. This is also true if there are any contraindications to NSAID use. Supportive or cognitive therapy can often help psychological stress that may be contributing to muscle spasm in headache, fibromyalgia, or back pain. Behavioral therapies likewise may reduce stress by providing distraction and giving the person greater control over pain (biofeedback, self-hypnosis, etc.). Remember that these therapies have no significant side effects, other than being somewhat expensive and time consuming, and they can lead to psychological growth and greater self-control. Of course, finding the right therapist is very important, since the effectiveness of these treatments depend heavily on having a good match between patient and counselor. Therefore, it is important to ask around for recommendations and investigate the reputation of the therapist before the first visit. For example, some counselors and psychologists are open to addressing and utilizing the spiritual strengths of the patient; others are not.

Don't use alcohol for pain relief, relaxation, or sleep. Stop smoking and other unhealthy habits that may contribute to physical deconditioning. Obtain a pet for company, although don't let it replace humans for companionship, and only take on the responsibility of pet ownership once you determine you will be able to properly care for your pet.

STEP 7: LOW-DOSE ANTIDEPRESSANTS, GABAPENTIN, AND MUSCLE RELAXANTS

If chronic pain persists despite these treatments, consider adjuvant therapies. Add a low dose of antidepressant to the current drug regimen to boost pain relief. For the younger person, I would suggest low-dose amitriptyline (10 to 25 mg) at bedtime. Amitriptyline is inexpensive, but it can have significant side effects (dry mouth, constipation, etc.). For the person over age sixty-five, I recommend nortrip-tyline (10 to 20 mg) at bedtime. Since higher doses are needed to treat depression, those recommended above assume that no depression is present, which is seldom the case. Venlafaxine (Effexor XR, 175 to 225 mg/day) is a good choice at any age, although it must be used cautiously in persons with high blood pressure. The dose noted is also close to that recommended for the treatment of depression.

If adding an antidepressant is ineffective or only partially effective, anticonvulsants may be tried (especially if the pain is neuropathic as seen in diabetes, trigeminal neuralgia, and certain chronic low back syndromes). Of the anticonvulsants, gabapentin (Neurontin, 300 to 1,800 mg/day) is least likely to interact with other medications and has the fewest side effects (although sedation can be a problem). Combining an antidepressant (such as venlafaxine) and gabapentin may be useful in certain cases.

If muscle spasm is contributing to the pain syndrome, then muscle relaxants such as cyclobenzaprine (Flexeril, 2.5 to 30 mg/day) or methocarbamol (Robaxin 750 to 4,500 mg/day) may help. Alterna-tively, benzodiazepines or antianxiety agents such as lorazepam (Ati-van, 0.25 to 2.0 mg/day) or clonazepam (Klonopin, 0.25 mg to 2.0 mg/day) may be tried. All of these drugs can cause significant seda-tion and may interfere with balance and coordination. Benzodiaz-epines may also be habit forming. Although typically used only in the short term, some persons have used these drugs over the long term with benefit.

As the number of drugs taken for pain begins to add up, the side ef-fects of these drugs also begin to accumulate. This is especially true for sedation, concentration difficulties, and problems with balance. Thus, it is probably at this point that one should seek help from a multidisciplinary team of pain experts.

STEP 8: TREATMENT IN A CHRONIC PAIN CLINIC

If chronic pain is moderate to severe in intensity and persists de-spite taking Steps 1 through 7 over three to six months, then serious consideration should be given to finding a chronic pain clinic nearby. In addition to the type of insurance coverage they accept, it is impor-tant to learn about the reputation of the pain clinic from people in the community, such as physicians, nurses, or social workers who have referred patients there and have received follow-up from those patients.

Ensure that a multidisciplinary team (physician who is an expert in pain therapies, clinical nurse specialist, psychologist, physical therapist, and occupational therapist, at minimum) is present in the clinic. Find out how quickly calls are returned by staff, how long it takes to schedule an appointment, and how often follow-up appointments are made. Are both inpatient and outpatient services available? What are the views of the physician and nurse toward surgery, use of narcotic pain relievers, and new advances in treatments for chronic pain? Is the patient considered a member of the treatment team, or do the health professionals make all the decisions? It is especially important to spend time with the clinic nurse, since this is the person likely to be seen during follow-up (more often than the physician).

Be sure to shop around to find a chronic pain clinic that will meet the patient's needs in a prompt, efficient, and comprehensive manner. It may be worth traveling a considerable distance if necessary for such services. An intensive chronic pain program may require the patient to remain at the treatment center eight hours a day, five days a week, for three to four weeks.[1]

STEP 9: SURGICAL THERAPIES AND OTHER MECHANICAL TREATMENTS

If there is a surgically correctable cause for the pain, then the appropriate procedures should be performed immediately after Step 1 has been taken. If there is no condition that is definitely treatable by surgery, then Steps 1 through 8 should be pursued first. If after following these steps the pain is not at least moderately controlled, then surgical procedures with a lower likelihood of success may be considered. Often, however, surgical procedures performed at this stage are associated with significant complications. If, however, there is at least a 50 percent chance that surgery will improve the problem, it may be worth taking the risk—especially if a skilled and highly reputable surgeon is willing to do the operation. New transcutaneous endoscopic approaches may soon reduce the complications seen with open surgical approaches, which could make this option more accept-able.

Injections of lidocaine, steroids, or other drugs into specific joints for relief of pain may provide at least short-term relief with relatively few complications if done correctly. Other mechanical treatments such as implantable spinal cord stimulators and implantable drug de-livery systems are less invasive than surgery, but are only effective in certain chronic pain conditions and in certain patients. Implantable devices should probably be considered before high-risk surgical pro-cedures are attempted. There are tests that can be done beforehand by the anesthesiologist or neurosurgeon to see whether a person is likely to benefit from such devices.

STEP 10: NARCOTIC ANALGESICS

This is the last step because of complications from the side effects and the problem of tolerance with opiates. Side effects of greatest worry are mental status changes (lethargy, sleepiness, decreased con-centration), balance problems (increased risk of falls and complica-tions of immobility), and nausea or constipation (particularly among persons taking multiple medications that may have constipating effects and older persons who suffer from bowel motility problems). With nar-cotics the possibility always exists that tolerance will develop, and higher and higher doses of the drug will be necessary to achieve the de-sired analgesic effect. Although this concern about addiction has been exaggerated in the past because of confusion between addiction and physical dependence, it still remains a worry. Furthermore, for certain pain syndromes such as headaches, regular use of opiates may even lead to analgesic rebound pain (see Chapter 13). Thus, the combina-tion of side effects and concern over developing tolerance make use of narcotics the last step in the treatment of nonmalignant chronic pain over the long term.

When it becomes necessary to use narcotic analgesics to relieve se-vere chronic pain that is resistant to other therapies and interferes with quality of life, which drug should be chosen? Based on my own clinical experience and that of other medical colleagues, I recom-mend oxycodone with either acetaminophen (e.g., Percocet, Tylox, etc.) or aspirin (Percodan, Endodan, etc.). The second drug of choice is probably long-acting morphine (MS Contin, Oramorph, etc.). Narcotic pain relievers should not be taken on an as-needed basis, but on a regular dosing schedule sufficient to relieve moderate to severe pain. Extra doses of medication may be required to treat breakthrough pain, but if such doses are necessary two or three times per day, then the amount of medication taken regularly should be increased. The goal is to achieve relief of severe pain with a minimum of side effects and to maximize physical, social, and occupational functioning. Even with use of narcotic pain relievers, rehabilitation is always the goal of chronic pain therapy.

SPECIAL SPIRITUAL STRATEGIES

Note that I have not included spiritual therapies as a separate step. This is because developing a spiritual attitude toward chronic pain and engaging in spiritual practices, as outlined in Chapter 14, is essential at every step to achieve maximum benefit. Here are some additional spiritual strategies that may help. Although many of these strategies are primarily directed toward Christians, persons from other religious backgrounds should consider adapting these practices to their own faiths.

Group Laying-on-of-Hands

Have two or three people commit to praying for the person in chronic pain. Have them meet with the person in pain and "lay hands on" that person. A light, gentle resting of the hand on the person's shoulder or upper back while saying a comforting and uplifting prayer can do wonders for the person's mood and feeling of being supported, and in some cases may even help to initiate neuroendocrine and immunological processes that speed healing or block pain.

Conduct a Spiritual Ritual

Consider conducting a religious ritual, with oil, incense, or perhaps Communion, during a healing service at church or synagogue. Because there are likely to be many persons in the congregation with some type of physical or emotional illness, such a healing service should be opened up to other people in addition to the person with chronic pain. In fact, there may be great benefit for chronic pain patients to pray for the health and personal needs of others as well; again, by providing comfort and healing to others, this may bring healing to the person in pain. Group rituals that involve worship and singing can be powerful strategies for producing pain relief and/or emotional comfort.

Try Spiritual Visualization

Progressive relaxation exercises or self-hypnosis may be used together with spiritual visualization to achieve pain relief. After entering a state of deep relaxation, visualize the painful body part. Then imagine God, Jesus, or the Holy Spirit coming into the room, laying His hands on the body part, and white light proceeding from His hands deep into the painful part. As this occurs, imagine a feeling of either warmth or coolness penetrating the painful area and displacing the pain. Repeat aloud over and over again a phrase, such as, "Jesus is bringing comfort and healing to my _____ (back, for example)." Take about fifteen to twenty minutes two or three times per day for this activity.

Perform Spiritual Acts of Mercy

Make a decision to do something three times each day to relieve the pain or suffering of someone else by praying for, listening to, or encouraging the person spiritually in some way. Visit someone in a nursing home or in the hospital, give someone a ride to church, call someone on the phone, or write someone a letter. Do this for thirty consecutive days and see how it affects you.

Start a Prayer Chain

Start a prayer chain of five to ten people with chronic pain. Call each of these people once a day for ten minutes to pray with, listen to, or encourage, and have them commit to do the same for one another. Depending on how many people are participating, adjust the frequency of calling so that each person in the prayer chain receives no more than three or four calls per day. Allow the prayer chain to continue with the original members for at least one month before opening it up to new members.

Find a Spiritual Role Model

Read the biographies of great spiritual people who have suffered physical pain, study their lives, and discover how they coped. Jesus is a good example for Christians. Others include the Christian martyrs (e.g., read the book *Jesus Freaks*,[2] and then look up some of the life stories the people discussed). Consider reading the lives of the saints (whether a person is from a Catholic background or not). The saints were often people struggling with great physical and emotional adversity who were able to overcome their problems through faith. Remember, though, that having a role model is different than worshiping someone.

Others

For those from a Christian background, consider taking time out after breakfast, after lunch, and before bedtime to place all your anger, discouragement, hopelessness, fear, worry, and lack of faith at the foot of the Cross. A simple religious ritual may assist this process. Do this for thirty consecutive days and see whether it makes a difference. Regardless of religious background, consider reading great classics such as *The Pilgrim's Progress*,[3] *Closer than a Brother*,[4] *Imitation of Christ*,[5] and others that stretch and extend faith.

SOURCES FOR FURTHER INFORMATION

For health professionals, religious professionals, or laypersons, the American Pain Society (APS) focuses on the diagnosis and appropriate treatment of people with chronic pain. The leadership of this group consists of basic clinical scientists, practicing clinicians, policy analysts, and others on the cutting edge of pain treatments. According to its Web site <www.ampainsoc.org>, the organization's purpose is to advance pain-related research, education, treatment, and professional practice. Begun in 1978, APS is a national chapter of the

International Association for the Study of Pain (IASP) and is reported to have more than 3,800 members, including physicians, nurses, psychologists, dentists, basic scientists, pharmacologists, therapists, and social workers. APS regularly holds pain management workshops and national symposia. It publishes *The Journal of Pain,* which had its first issue in early 2000; prior to that, APS published a newsletter, *Pain Forum,* which the journal replaced. For those wishing for more information about recent developments in the treatment of pain, contact APS by e-mail <info@ampainsoc.org>, regular mail (at 4700 W. Lake Avenue, Glenview, Illinois 60025), or by telephone (847-375-4715).

Besides *The Journal of Pain,* APS has several other publications. *APS Bulletin*[6] is a bimonthly publication offering articles on clinical, research, and organizational news concerning the treatment of pain, as well as a calendar of special events; this can be viewed online from the APS Web site. *Managed Care and Pain*[7] is a periodical that provides information to help pain specialists and managed care decision makers develop chronic pain programs that are high quality and cost effective. *Guidelines for the Management of Acute and Chronic Pain in Sickle-Cell Disease*[8] is a book designed to help physicians, nurses, pharmacists, and other health care professionals manage the pain experienced by those with sickle-cell disease. *Principles of Analgesic Use in the Treatment of Acute Pain and Cancer Pain*[9] is a practical guide, now in its fourth edition, that helps clinicians select the appropriate drug, dose, and route for treating pain. It also describes how to best treat breakthrough pain, while at the same time minimizing side effects. This guide, claimed to be an ideal resource for medical and nursing students, is available for a minimal cost (four dollars for members, seven dollars for nonmembers). All of these publications can be ordered through the APS Web site.

Duke University Medical Center (DUMC) has a Pain and Palliative Care Program <www.pain.mc.duke.edu>. This program began monitoring pain in all inpatients at DUMC in 1997. It has a single telephone number that both patients and referring physicians can call for pain-related appointments (919-684-PAIN). The Web site has comprehensive information on pain medications (costs, doses, precautions, information about effective administration), complementary therapies, suggestions for managing pain in all ages, and ten ways parents can help ease pain in children. They also distribute pocket-sized reference cards that include six pain assessment scales for adults, children, and infants, medication guidelines, an opiate conversion table, a palliative care program quick reference guide, and information about side effects of treatments. These cards can be ordered online at the Web site (click on Duke Pain Initiative, then on Request Supplies).

Finally, The Haworth Press publishes the *Journal of Musculoskeletal Pain* and the *Journal of Pain and Palliative Care in Pharmacotherapy,* which provides a wealth of practical information about treatments for pain.

SUMMARY AND CONCLUSIONS

Those who experience chronic pain have many things they can do to slay the relentless giant that has imprisoned them. If they cannot slay the giant, they can at least live with him in a tolerable relationship. Following a comprehensive medical and surgical evaluation, simple drug and nondrug treatments with minimal side effects and cost should be considered. If these are ineffective or only partially effective, additional steps should be taken as outlined, proceeding all the way to long-term use of narcotic analgesics as necessary. The addition of spiritual strategies at each step provides additional hope that a long-term relationship with chronic pain will not only be tolerable but have meaning and purpose and help to achieve our ultimate goals in both this life and perhaps the next one as well—deeper and more fulfilling relationships with God, with our neighbors, and with ourselves.

Appendix I

Healing Scriptures
for Those in Chronic Pain

My son, pay attention to what I say; listen closely to my *words*.
Do not let them out of your sight, keep them within your heart;
for they are *life* to those who find them and *health* to a man's *whole body*.

Proverbs 4:20-22

A systematic computer search of the Bible (NIV and KJV) reveals many Scriptures on suffering and healing. They are presented here in chronological order. A total of twenty-seven on suffering and, interestingly, sixty on healing were found. These Scriptures may be repeated silently or read out loud. Each one should be concentrated and meditated upon, allowing the healing words to deeply infuse the mind, body, and spirit. They are as powerful a medicine as the drugs listed in Appendix II, and may be used together with those drugs to enhance analgesic effects.

SCRIPTURES CONCERNING SUFFERING AND PAIN

The LORD said, "I have indeed seen the misery of my people in Egypt.
I have heard them crying out because of their slave drivers [pain],
    and I am concerned about their suffering.
So I have come down to rescue them from the hand of the Egyptians
    and to bring them up out of that land into a good and spacious land,
    a land flowing with milk and honey . . ."

Exodus 3:7-8

"Not so, my lord," Hannah replied,
"I am a woman who is deeply troubled.
I have not been drinking wine or beer;

I was pouring out my soul to the LORD.
Do not take your servant for a wicked woman;
I have been praying here out of my great anguish and grief."
[Pain often prompts us to turn to God in prayer]

1 Samuel 1:15-16

But those who suffer he delivers in their suffering;
he speaks to them in their affliction.

Job 36:15

Be merciful to me, LORD, for I am faint;
    O LORD, heal me, for my bones are in agony.
My soul is in anguish.
How long, O LORD, how long?

Psalm 6:2-3

For he has not despised or disdained
    the suffering of the afflicted one;
he has not hidden his face from him
    but has listened to his cry for help.

Psalm 22:24

The troubles of my heart have multiplied;
    free me from my anguish.
Look upon my affliction and my distress
    and take away all my sins . . .
Guard my life and rescue me;
    let me not be put to shame,
    for I take refuge in you.
May integrity and uprightness protect me,
    because my hope is in you.

Psalm 25:17-18, 20-21

Be merciful to me, O LORD, for I am in distress;
    my eyes grow weak with sorrow,
    my soul and my body with grief.
My life is consumed by anguish
    and my years by groaning;
my strength fails because of my affliction,
    and my bones grow weak.

Psalm 31:9-10

I am in pain and distress;
   may your salvation, O God, protect me.
I will praise God's name in song
   and glorify him with thanksgiving.

                             Psalm 69:29-30

The cords of death entangled me,
   the anguish of the grave came upon me;
   I was overcome by trouble and sorrow.
But then I called on the name of the LORD:
  "O LORD, save me!"

                             Psalm 116:3-4

Remember your word to your servant,
   for you have given me hope.
My comfort in my suffering is this:
   Your promise preserves my life.
The arrogant mock me without restraint,
   but I do not turn from your law.
I remember your ancient laws, O LORD,
and I find comfort in them.

                             Psalm 119:49-52

Look upon my suffering and deliver me,
   for I have not forgotten your law.

                             Psalm 119:153

You restored me to health
   and let me live.
Surely it was for my benefit
   that I suffered such anguish.

                             Isaiah 38:16-17

He [Christ] was despised and rejected by men,
a man of sorrows, and familiar with suffering.

                             Isaiah 53:3

Is there no balm in Gilead?
    Is there no physician there?
Why then is there no healing
    for the wound of my people? . . .
Therefore this is what the LORD Almighty says:
"See, I will refine and test them . . ."

Jeremiah 8:22, 9:7

I sat alone because your hand was on me
    and you had filled me with indignation.
Why is my pain unending
    and my wound grievous and incurable?
Will you be to me like a deceptive brook,
    like a spring that fails?
Therefore this is what the LORD says:
"If you repent, I will restore you
    that you may serve me;
if you utter worthy, not worthless, words,
    you will be my spokesman."

Jeremiah 15:17-19

And being in anguish, he [Jesus] prayed more earnestly,
and his sweat was like drops of blood falling to the ground.

Luke 22:44

The apostles left the Sanhedrin, rejoicing
because they had been counted worthy of suffering disgrace for the
    Name.

Acts 5:41

And we rejoice in the hope of the glory of God.
Not only so, but we also rejoice in our sufferings,
because we know that suffering produces perseverance;
perseverance, character; and character, hope.
And hope does not disappoint us,
because God has poured out his love into our hearts
by the Holy Spirit . . .

Romans 5:2-5

No, in all these things [including chronic pain]
we are more than conquerors
through him who loved us.

Romans 8:37

You became imitators of us and of the Lord;
in spite of severe suffering, you welcomed the message [of the
    Gospel]
with the joy given by the Holy Spirit.
And so you became a model to all the believers . . .

1 Thessalonians 1:6-7

But join with me in suffering for the gospel,
by the power of God, who has saved us
and called us to a holy life—
not because of anything we have done
but because of his own purpose and grace.

2 Timothy 1:8-9

This is my gospel, for which I am suffering
even to the point of being chained like a criminal.
But God's word is not chained.
Therefore I endure everything for the sake of the elect,
that they too may obtain the salvation that is in Christ Jesus,
with eternal glory.

2 Timothy 2:8-10

In bringing many sons to glory, it was fitting that God,
for whom and through whom everything exists,
should make the author of their salvation perfect through suffering.
Both the one who makes men holy and those who are made holy
are of the same family.
So Jesus is not ashamed to call them brothers.

Hebrews 2:10-11

Brothers, as an example of patience in the face of suffering,
take the prophets who spoke in the name of the Lord.
As you know, we consider blessed those who have persevered.

You have heard of Job's perseverance
and have seen what the Lord finally brought about.
The Lord is full of compassion and mercy.

James 5:10-11

For it is commendable
if a man bears up under the pain of unjust suffering
because he is conscious of God.

1 Peter 2:19

Dear friends, do not be surprised at the painful trial you are suffering,
as though something strange were happening to you.
But rejoice that you participate in the sufferings of Christ,
so that you may be overjoyed when his glory is revealed.
[Whether persecutions are external or internal makes little difference.
Today, internal persecutions and physical pain often take the place of
the external persecutions that Jesus' disciples had to face. Suffering
with an attitude toward participating in the sufferings of Christ will
achieve the same result as Jesus' disciples persistence in testifying accomplished.]

1 Peter 4:12-13

And I heard a loud voice from the throne saying,
"Now the dwelling of God is with men, and he will live with them.
They will be his people,
and God himself will be with them and be their God.
He will wipe every tear from their eyes.
There will be no more death or mourning or crying or pain,
for the old order of things has passed away."

Revelation 21:3-4

SCRIPTURES CONCERNING HEALING

See now that I, *even* I, *am* he,
and *there is* no god with me:
I kill, and I make alive;
I wound, and I heal . . .

Deuteronomy 32:39 (KJV)[2]

Thus saith the LORD, the God of David thy father,
I have heard thy prayer, I have seen thy tears:
behold, I will heal thee . . .

                                  2 Kings 20:5 (KJV)

O LORD my God, I called to you for help
and you healed me.

                                  Psalm 30:2

I said, LORD, be merciful unto me: heal my soul . . .

                                  Psalm 41:4 (KJV)

Then they cried to the LORD in their trouble,
   and he saved them from their distress.
He sent forth his word and healed them . . .

                                  Psalm 107:19-20

Do not be wise in your own eyes;
   fear the LORD and shun evil.
This will bring health to your body
 and nourishment to your bones.

                                  Proverbs 3:7

Reckless words pierce like a sword,
but the tongue of the wise brings healing.

                                  Proverbs 12:18

The tongue that brings healing is a tree of life,
but a deceitful tongue crushes the spirit.

                                  Proverbs 15:4

A cheerful look brings joy to the heart,
and good news gives health to the bones.

                                  Proverbs 15:30

Pleasant words are a honeycomb,
sweet to the soul and healing to the bones.

                                                    Proverbs 16:24

Surely he took up our infirmities
    and carried our sorrows,
yet we considered him stricken by God,
    smitten by him, and afflicted.
But he was pierced for our transgressions,
    he was crushed for our iniquities;
the punishment that brought us peace was upon him,
    and *by his wounds we are healed.*

                                                    Isaiah 53:4-5

I have seen his ways, and will heal him:
I will lead him also,
and restore comforts unto him and to his mourners.
I create the fruit of the lips;
Peace, peace to *him that is* far off,
and to *him that is* near, saith the LORD;
and I will heal him.

                                              Isaiah 57:18-19 (KJV)

Is it not to share your food with the hungry
    and to provide the poor wanderer with shelter—
when you see the naked, to clothe him,
    and not to turn away from your own flesh and blood?
Then your light will break forth like the dawn,
    and your healing will quickly appear . . .

                                                    Isaiah 58:7-8

Heal me, O LORD, and I will be healed;
    save me and I will be saved,
for you are the one I praise.

                                                    Jeremiah 17:14

"But I will restore you to health
    and heal your wounds,"
declares the LORD . . .

                                                    Jeremiah 30:17

. . . I will heal my people
and will let them enjoy abundant peace and security.

Jeremiah 33:6

Come, and let us return unto the LORD:
for he hath torn, and he will heal us;
he hath smitten, and he will bind us up.

Hosea 6:1 (KJV)

It was I [the Lord] who taught Ephraim to walk,
    taking them by the arms;
but they did not realize
    it was I who healed them.

Hosea 11:3

But for you who revere my name,
the sun of righteousness will rise with healing in its wings.
And you will go out and leap like calves released from the stall.

Malachi 4:2

Jesus went throughout Galilee, teaching in their synagogues,
preaching the good news of the kingdom,
and healing every disease and sickness among the people.
News about him spread all over Syria,
and people brought to him all who were ill with various diseases,
those suffering severe pain, the demon-possessed, those having
    seizures, and the paralyzed, and he healed them.

Matthew 4:23-24

"Lord," he said, "my servant lies at home paralyzed and in terrible
    suffering."
Jesus said to him, "I will go and heal him."

Matthew 8:6-7

When evening came, many who were demon-possessed were brought
    to him,
and he drove out the spirits with a word and healed all the sick.
This was to fulfill what was spoken through the prophet Isaiah:
"He took up our infirmities and carried our diseases."

Matthew 8:16-17

Just then a woman who had been subject to bleeding for twelve years
came up behind him and touched the edge of his cloak.
She said to herself, "If I only touch his cloak, I will be healed."
Jesus turned and saw her. "Take heart, daughter," he said,
"your faith has healed you."
And the woman was healed from that moment.

Matthew 9:20-21

Jesus went through all the towns and villages,
teaching in their synagogues, preaching the good news of the kingdom
and healing every disease and sickness.

Matthew 9:35

And when he had called unto *him* his twelve disciples,
he gave them power *against* unclean spirits, to cast them out,
and to heal all manner of sickness and all manner of disease.

Matthew 10:1 (KJV)

When Jesus landed and saw a large crowd,
he had compassion on them and healed their sick.

Matthew 14:14

People brought all their sick to him
and begged him to let the sick just touch the edge of his cloak,
and all who touched him were healed.

Matthew 14:35-36

Great crowds came to him, bringing the lame,
the blind, the crippled, the mute and many others,
and laid them at his feet;
and he healed them.

Matthew 15:30

When Jesus had finished saying these things,
he left Galilee and went into the region of Judea to the
    other side of the Jordan.
Large crowds followed him,
and he healed them there.

Matthew 19:1-2

The blind and the lame came to him at the temple,
and he healed them.

Matthew 21:14

The whole town gathered at the door,
and Jesus healed many who had various diseases.

Mark 1:33-34

For he had healed many,
so that those with diseases were pushing forward to touch him.

Mark 3:10

And he ordained twelve, that they should be with him,
and that he might send them forth to preach,
And to have power to heal sicknesses, and to cast out devils [pain] . . .

Mark 3:14-15 (KJV)

He said to her, "Daughter, your faith has healed you.
Go in peace and be freed from your suffering."

Mark 5:34

They went out and preached that people should repent.
They drove out many demons
and anointed many sick people with oil and healed them.

Mark 6:12-13

They begged him to let them touch even the edge of his cloak,
and all who touched him were healed.

Mark 6:56

"Go," said Jesus, "your faith has healed you."
Immediately he received his sight and followed Jesus along the road.

Mark 10:52

. . . the people brought to Jesus all who had various kinds of sickness,
and laying his hands on each one, he healed them.

Luke 4:40

Yet the news about him spread all the more,
so that crowds of people came to hear him
and to be healed of their sicknesses.

Luke 5:15

A large crowd of his disciples was there
and a great number of people from all over Judea,
from Jerusalem, and from the coast of Tyre and Sidon,
who had come to hear him and to be healed of their diseases.

Luke 6:17-18

Those troubled by evil spirits were cured,
and the people all tried to touch him,
because power was coming from him and healing them all.

Luke 6:18-19

Hearing this, Jesus said to Jairus, "Don't be afraid;
just believe, and she will be healed."

Luke 8:50

And he sent them to preach the kingdom of God,
and to heal the sick.

Luke 9:2 (KJV)

So they [Jesus' twelve disciples] set out and went from village
    to village,
preaching the gospel and healing people everywhere.

Luke 9:6

. . . but the crowds learned about it and followed him.
He welcomed them and spoke to them about the kingdom of God,
and healed those who needed healing.

Luke 9:11

Even while the boy was coming,
the demon threw him to the ground in a convulsion.
But Jesus rebuked the evil spirit,
healed the boy and gave him back to his father.

Luke 9:42

So taking hold of the man, he healed him and sent him away.

Luke 14:4

Jesus said to him, "Receive your sight; your faith has healed you."

Luke 18:4

But Jesus answered, "No more of this!"
And he touched the man's ear and healed him.

Luke 22:51

The thief comes only to steal and kill and destroy;
I have come that they may have life,
and have it to the full [abundantly, in KJV].

John 10:10

By faith in the name of Jesus,
this man whom you see and know was made strong.
It is Jesus' name and the faith that comes through him
that has given this complete healing to him . . .

Acts 3:16

Crowds gathered also from the towns around Jerusalem [to hear Peter
    talk],
bringing their sick and those tormented by evil spirits,
and all of them were healed.

Acts 5:16

When the crowds heard Philip and saw the miraculous signs he did,
they all paid close attention to what he said.
With shrieks, evil spirits came out of many,
and many paralytics and cripples were healed.

Acts 8:6-7

That *word, I* say, ye know,
which was published throughout all Judaea,
and began from Galilee, after the baptism which John preached;
How God anointed Jesus of Nazareth with the Holy Ghost
    and with power:
who went about doing good,

and healing all that were oppressed of the devil;
for God was with him.

Acts 10:37-38 (KJV)

He listened to Paul as he was speaking.
Paul looked directly at him, saw that he had faith to be healed
and called out, "Stand up on your feet!"
At that, the man jumped up and began to walk.

Acts 14:9-10

His father was sick in bed, suffering from fever and dysentery.
Paul went in to see him and, after prayer,
placed his hands on him and healed him.
When this had happened, the rest of the sick on the island came
    and were cured.

Acts 28:8-9

Therefore, strengthen your feeble arms and weak knees.
"Make level paths for your feet,"
so that the lame may not be disabled, but rather healed.

Hebrews 12:12-13

Therefore confess your sins to each other
and pray for each other so that you may be healed.
The prayer of a righteous man is powerful and effective.

James 5:16

He himself bore our sins in his body on the tree,
so that we might die to sins and live for righteousness;
by his wounds you have been healed.

1 Peter 2:24

Dear friend, I pray that you may enjoy good health
and that all may go well with you,
even as your soul is getting along well.

3 John 1:2

Appendix II

Medications for Pain and Managing Side Effects

Appendix II contains three tables. Table II.1 examines nonnarcotic medicine for mild to moderately intense chronic pain. Table II.2 describes narcotic or opium-derived medications useful for moderate to severe chronic pain. Table II.3 discusses treatments for side effects of narcotic pain relievers.

TABLE II.1. Nonnarcotic Analgesics for Mild to Moderate Chronic Pain

Name	Preparation	Dose (adult)	Comments and Precautions
Acetaminophen/OTC** (Tylenol*)	Tablet or capsule: 325 mg (regular) 500 mg (extra-strength)	325 to 1,000 mg every 4-8 hours (not to exceed 4,000 mg/day for short-term use, 3,200 mg/d for chronic use, or 2,400 mg/d if debilitated, alcoholic, or malnourished)	Long-term use is usually safe, but need to monitor liver and kidney function. Few interactions with other drugs. For most persons, this is the safest and first choice for treatment of pain. Need to take on a regular scheduled basis to maximize benefit, rather than only as needed.
Nonsteroidal Anti-Inflammatory Drugs (NSAIDs)			
Aspirin/OTC (Bufferin*, Ascriptin* contain buffering agents that help to relieve stomach irritation; also Ecotrin* is form of coated	Tablet: 325 mg (regular) 80 mg (baby aspirin)	650 mg every 4-6 hours (until ears ring or 3,900 mg/d max)	Increases bleeding; may cause peptic ulcer; allergic reactions; may affect kidney function.

279

Name	Preparation	Dose (adult)	Comments and Precautions
aspirin with less stomach irritation)			
Other NSAIDs: ibuprofen/OTC (Advil*, Motrin*), naproxen/OTC (Aleve*, Naprosyn*), indomethacin (Indocin*), endolac (Lodine*), ketorolac (Toradol*), others	Tablet or capsule: preparations vary Injection (IV): ketorolac	Doses vary	Increases bleeding; may cause peptic ulcer; allergic reactions; may affect kidney and liver function.
COX-2 Inhibitors			
Celecoxib (Celebrex*)	Capsule: 100 mg, 200 mg	50 to 200 mg every 12 hours	Minimal gastrointestinal side effects (peptic ulcer); increases bleeding; may affect kidney and liver function; contraindicated if sulfonamide (sulfa) allergy.
Rofecoxib (Vioxx*)	Tablet: 12.5 mg, 25 mg Solution: 25 mg/ml	12.5 or 25 mg every 12 hours	Minimal gastrointestinal side effects (peptic ulcer); increases bleeding; may affect kidney function.
Drug Combinations			
Excedrin Migraine*/ OTC	Tablet: 250-500 mg acetaminophen, 250-500 mg aspirin and 32-65 mg caffeine	Two tablets every 6 hours as needed	Same cautions as for acetaminophen and aspirin. Caffeine may cause insomnia.
Anacin*/OTC	Tablet: 400 mg aspirin and 32 mg caffeine (500 mg aspirin in Extra-Strength Anacin*)	2 tablets every 6 hours as needed	Same precautions as for aspirin; caffeine may cause insomnia.
BC* tablets or powder/ OTC	Tablet: 325 mg aspirin, 16 mg caffeine, and 195 mg salicylamide	2 tablets every 6 hours as needed	Same precautions as for aspirin; caffeine may cause insomnia.

Name	Preparation	Dose (adult)	Comments and Precautions
Muscle Relaxants			
Cyclobenzaprine (Flexeril*) (used in combination with analgesics)	Tablet: 10 mg	Dose varies from 2.5 mg/d (¼ tablet at bedtime) to 40 mg/d (10 mg every 6-8 hours)	Side effects and cautions are similar to those for tricyclic antidepressants such as amitriptyline (see following). Sedation can be a problem, so avoid when driving.
Methocarbamol (Robaxin*) (used in combination with analgesics)	Tablet: 1,500 mg	1,500 mg every 6 hours	Should avoid use in elderly due to anticholinergic side effects. Sedation can be a problem. Do not use in persons with seizure disorder or kidney disease.
Anti-Inflammatory			
Prednisone / Cortisol (Deltasone* or Orasone*)	Tablet: 1 mg, 2.5 mg, 5 mg, 10 mg, 20 mg, 50 mg Oral solution: 5 mg/5 cc's	5 to 60 mg/day	Powerful anti-inflammatory drug with numerous side effects: mood alteration, loss of bone mass, thinning of skin, peptic ulcers, muscle weakness, fluid retention, weight gain, cataracts, increased infection.
Methotrexate (Rheumatrex*)	Tablet: 2.5 mg Solution for injection: (25 mg/ml) Powder for injection (1 to 50 mg)	5 to 25 mg as single weekly dose either orally, intra-muscular, or intravenously	Antimetabolite and chemo-therapeutic drug used to treat rheumatoid arthritis; causes immunosuppression and may have liver and serious other organ toxicity; requires monitoring with liver biopsies.
Infliximab (anti-tumor necrosis factor [TNF] antibody)	IV solution	3 mg/kg to 10 mg/kg every 4-8 weeks	Targets the key inflammatory cytokine TNF; for use in rheumatoid arthritis. Increased risk of infection due to suppression of immune system.
Anticonvulsants			
Carbamazepine (Tegretol*)	Tablet: 100, 200 mg; 200-400 mg extended	Oral preparation 100 mg twice a	Has many side effects (SEs), including serious ones

Name	Preparation	Dose (adult)	Comments and Precautions
(for trigeminal or post-herpetic neuralgia, multiple sclerosis, diabetic neuropathy, postamputation or postlaminectomy)	release	day to 300 mg four times a day	involving the blood, and interacts with other medications.
Gabapentin (Neurontin*) (used in combination with analgesics)	Capsules: 100, 300, 400 mg	Oral preparation 100 mg three times a day to 600 mg three times a day (do not exceed 3,600 mg/day)	Has fewer SEs than carbamezepine and relatively safe, although can produce excessive sedation; interacts with few medicines.

Antidepressants

Name	Preparation	Dose (adult)	Comments and Precautions
Amitriptyline (Elavil*) (typically used in combination with other pain medicines)	Tablet: 10, 25, 50, 75, 100, 150 mg	10-25 mg/day for pain; 150-300 mg/day for depression Take at bedtime to help with sleep and reduce daytime grogginess.	SEs may include dry mouth, sedation, difficulty urinating, weight gain, constipation; should not be used in patients with certain types of glaucoma, those who have heart block or following heart attack, those who are taking certain kinds of medication (monoamine oxidase inhibitors [MAOIs]), or those with difficulty urinating due to prostate or other problems. See *Physician's Desk Reference* (PDR) for full list of cautions and contraindications.
Nortriptyline (Pamelor*) (typically used in combination with other pain medicines)	Capsule: 10, 25, 50, 75 mg	10-25 mg/day for pain; 50-125 mg/day for depression Take at bedtime to help sleep.	Same as for amitriptyline, but not as severe; safer for use in older adults.
Doxepin (Sinequan*)	Capsule:10, 25, 50 mg	10-25 mg/day for pain; 150-	Same as for amitriptyline.

Name	Preparation	Dose (adult)	Comments and Precautions
(typically used in combination with other pain medicines)		300 mg/day for depression Take at bedtime to help sleep.	
Fluoxetine (Prozac*) and other selective serotonin reuptake inhibitors (SSRIs)	Capsule: 10, 20 mg	Not very effective for pain alone; 10-40 mg/day for depression	Drowsiness or insomnia, nausea, sexual dysfunction, and nervousness are SEs that may or may not occur; should not be used with MAOIs.
Antianxiety Drugs			
Lorazepam (Ativan*)	Tablet: 0.5, 1.0, and 2.0 mg	Dose: 0.5 to 2.0 mg every 6 to 24 hours (usual	Caution since may be habit forming; can cause excessive sedation and interfere with
May help decrease threshold at which pain is experienced	Liquid: 2 mg/cc Parenteral: 2 mg/cc and 4 mg/cc	dose is 0.5 to 1.0 mg once or twice daily)	concentration, memory, or balance.
Others			
Topical lidocaine patch	Patch	Leave on for 12 hours at night and take off	Effective for postherpetic neuralgia, diabetic neuropathy.
Topical EMLA* with patch (lidocaine and prilocaine combo)		during daytime	Costly ($100 for 30 patches); rash occurs in 25 percent of cases.
Lidocaine 2.5 percent and prilocaine 2.5 percent cream (EMLA*)	Cream (5 gm and 30 gm tubes) Apply 1 hour before minor procedures, 2 hours before major	Apply cream as thick layer over 2×2 inch area. Cover with cellophane wrap.	Use for pain coming from skin conditions; use only on dermal skin; contraindicated in methemoglobinemia.
Capsaicin (Capzasin-P*, Eucalyptamint* 2000, Icy Hot*, Ben-Gay*, others) (major ingredient is hot chile pepper). Used for the treatment of mild pain or moderate pain associated with rheumatoid arthritis or osteoarthritis. (OTC)	Cream; apply sparingly and rub well into affected area until little or no cream is left on the surface of the skin.	Topical dosage: apply capsaicin 0.025 percent or 0.075 percent topically to painful joints 4 times per day. Duration of action is 4-6 hours; pain relief usually	Wash hands with soap after applying to avoid getting into eyes or other sensitive areas; if used on arthritic hands, leave on for at least 30 minutes after application. Do not apply to irritated or broken skin, or to areas with skin abrasion. Do not use with a heating pad or after strenuous exercise. If condition worsens

Name	Preparation	Dose (adult)	Comments and Precautions
		noted within 2 weeks of therapy	or persists more than 7 days, or clears up and occurs again within a few days, capsaicin therapy should be discontinued. Do not use if sensitive to hot peppers.
Chondroitin-glucosamine combination/OTC (Cortaflex*, Cosamin*, Osteo-Bi-Flex*) (categorized as a dietary supplement; used for osteoarthritis)	Capsules (Cosamin*-DS): 500 mg glucosamine HCL and 400 mg chondroitin sulfate. Same contents for Osteo-Bi-Flex* Maximum Strength tablet or softgel.	Take 3 capsules/day (2 in morning and 1 in evening) for first 2 months; then may reduce dose to that which maintains comfort.	Chondroitin may inhibit the enzymes that destroy cartilage; glucosamine may enhance the cartilage repair process. Drowsiness reported which may affect driving or operating machinery. GI symptoms may occur. Use cautiously in cardiac disease. Data on effectiveness are limited.
Glucosamine (alone)	Capsules: 500 mg	Take 3 capsules/day	This substance is relatively safe, although same precautions as above for the combination of chondroitin-glucosamine.

*Brand name
**OTC = over-the-counter (nonprescription) medication

TABLE II.2. Narcotic Analgesics for Moderate to Severe Chronic Pain

Name	Preparation	Dose / Morphine Equivalent	Comments and Precautions
Opioids—Strong			
Morphine sulfate (MS) (morphine) Immediate Release (MSIR*, Roxanol*)	MSIR or Roxanol* Tablet: 10 mg, 15 mg, 30 mg; Capsule: 15 mg MSIR oral solution: 10 mg/5 cc or 20 mg/5cc;	10-30 mg every 3-4 hours (oral) 2-10 mg every 2-4 hours (parenteral**)	MS used as standard of comparison for all opioid (narcotic) pain relievers Common side effects: somnolence (excessive

Name	Preparation	Dose / Morphine Equivalent	Comments and Precautions
Continuous Release (MS Contin*, Oramorph*)	or 2, 4, or 20 mg/cc		sleeping), trouble concentrating, constipation, nausea and vomiting, itching, respiratory depression (slowed breathing)
	Roxanol* suppository: 5 mg, 10 mg, 20 mg, 30 mg	No maximum dose	
	Parenteral MSIR*: 0.5 25.0 mg/cc	Peak effect in one hour	May be habit forming
	MS Contin* Tablet: 15 mg, 30 mg, 60 mg, 100 mg, 200 mg		Oral solution contains alcohol
			MS Contin* tablets not to be cut, crushed, or chewed
	Sustained Release Capsule: 20 mg, 50 mg, 100 mg		
Fentanyl (Duragesic*)	Transdermal patch: 10 cm^2 (25 mcg/hr) 20 cm^2 (50 mcg/hr) 30 cm^2 (75 mcg/hr) 40 cm^2 (100 mcg/hr)	100 mcg fentanyl = 30 mg oral MS; 25 mcg/hr fentanyl = 2.5 mg IV MS/hr	Only used in opioid-tolerant patients
		IV: 0.25-1 mcg/kg	Side effects: see morphine
	Parenteral solution (50 mcg/ml)	Every 10 minutes for procedures	May be habit forming
Hydromorphone (Dilaudid*)	Tablet: 1 mg, 2 mg, 3 mg, 4 mg, and 8 mg	7.5 mg oral = 30 mg oral MS	Duration of action is slightly shorter than morphine.
	Oral liquid: 1 mg/cc	1.5 mg parenteral = 10 mg parenteral MS	Side effects: see morphine
	Parenteral solution: 1 mg/cc to 10 mg/cc	Oral dose 1-4 mg every 2-6 hours;	May be habit forming
	Rectal suppository: 3 mg	IV dose 0.5-2 mg every 2-6 hours	

Name	Preparation	Dose / Morphine Equivalent	Comments and Precautions
Meperidine HCL (Demerol*) (limited to pain after surgery or painful diagnostic procedures; use only short term)	Tablet: 50 mg, 100 mg Syrup: 50 mg/5 cc's Parenteral: 10 to 100 mg/cc	300 mg oral = 30 mg oral MS (50-150 mg every 3-4 hours) 100 mg parenteral = 10 mg parenteral MS	Shorter duration than morphine Side effects: see morphine; also avoid use in renal failure or history of seizures; interacts negatively with St. John's wort; don't use with Phenergan.* May be habit forming
Heroin, diamorphine HCL (not available in United States)	Parenteral only	4-5 mg parenteral = 10 mg parenteral MS	Shorter duration than morphine
Methadone HCL (Dolphine*) (limited to those with severe chronic pain)	Tablet: 5 mg, 10 mg, 40 mg Oral solution: 1-10 mg/cc Parenteral: 10 mg/cc	30 mg oral = 30 mg oral MS 10 mg parenteral = 10 mg parenteral MS (2.5-10 mg parenteral every 3-4 hours) Reduce dose if renal impairment present	Same duration as morphine Accumulates with repeated dosing, requiring decreased dose on days 2-5; peak effect seen in 4-10 days; takes 4-10 days to eliminate from body Side effects: see morphine May be habit forming

Opioids—Moderate

Name	Preparation	Dose / Morphine Equivalent	Comments and Precautions
Hydrocodone bitartrate (with acetaminophen: Lorcet,* Lortab*, Vicodin)*	Tablet: 5/500 (5 mg hydrocodone with 500 mg acetaminophen) Elixir: 5 or 7.5/500 per 15 cc (Lortab elixir)	30 mg hydrocodone = 30 mg oral MS (1 or 2 tablets every 4-6 hours)	Only in the oral form Side effects: see morphine May be habit forming
Hydrocodone	Tablet: 5/500	Same as above	Same as above

Name	Preparation	Dose / Morphine Equivalent	Comments and Precautions
bitartrate (with aspirin: Azdone)	(5 mg hydrocodone with 500 mg aspirin)		
Oxycodone (with acetaminophen: Percocet, Tylox, Roxilox, Endocet)	Tablet: 5/325 (Percocet), 5/500 (Roxicet) Capsule:5/500 (Tylox) Oral solution: 5/325 per 5 cc	20 mg oxycodone = 30 mg oral MS (1 or 2 tablets every 4-6 hours)	Only in the oral form Side effects: see morphine May be habit forming
	(5 mg oxycodone with 325 or 500 mg acetaminophen)		
Oxycodone (with aspirin: Percodan)	Tablet: 5/325 (5 mg oxycodone with 325 mg aspirin)	Same as above	Same as above
Pentazocine HCL (with aspirin: Talwin)	Tablet: 12.5/325 (12.5 mg pentazocine with 325 mg aspirin)	60 mg oral Pentazocine = 30 mg oral MS	Shorter duration than morphine
		(25 mg oral every 6-8 hours)	Side effects: see morphine
		60 mg parenteral = 10 mg parenteral MS	May be habit forming

Opioids—Milder

Name	Preparation	Dose / Morphine Equivalent	Comments and Precautions
Propoxyphene napsylate (with acetaminophen: Darvocet-N*)	Tablet: Darvocet N-50 has 50 mg propoxyphene and 325 mg acetaminophen; Darvocet N100 has 100 mg propoxyphene and 650 mg acetaminophen.	500 mg oral propoxyphene = 30 mg oral MS (100 mg propoxyphene napsylate every 4 hours, not to exceed 600 mg/day)	Only in the oral form Side effects: see morphine May be habit forming
Propoxyphene HCL (with aspirin: Darvon*)	Capsule: Darvon* has 65 mg propoxyphene HCL, 389 mg aspirin, and 32 mg caffeine	325 mg propoxy-Aphene HCL = 30 mg oral MS	Only in the oral form Side effects: see morphine
(with acetaminophen: Wygesic*)	Wygesic* has 65 mg propoxyphene and 650 mg acetaminophen	(65 mg propoxyphene HCL every 4-6 hours, not to exceed 390/day, or 6 capsules/day)	May be habit forming

Name	Preparation	Dose / Morphine Equivalent	Comments and Precautions
Codeine (with acetaminophen: Tylenol* with codeine)	Tablet: 15 mg, 30 mg, 60 mg, each with 300 mg acetaminophen (No. 2, No. 3, No. 4, respectively) Elixir: 12 mg codeine and 120 mg aceta- minophen per 5 cc's in 7 percent alcohol	150 mg oral codeine = 30 mg oral MS (15-60 mg codeine every 4 hours, not to exceed 360 mg/day; acetaminophen not to exceed 4,000 mg/day)	Only in the oral form Side effects: see morphine May be habit forming
Codeine (with aspirin: Emperin* with codeine)	Tablet: 15 mg, 30 mg, 60 mg, each with 325 mg aspirin (No. 2, No. 3, No. 4, respectively)	150 mg oral codeine = 30 mg oral MS (15-60 mg codeine every 4 hours, not to exceed 360 mg/day)	Only in the oral form Side effects: see morphine May be habit forming
Tramadol HCL (Ultram*)	Tablet: 50 mg (considered nonnarcotic by FDA but acts on opioid receptors)	300 mg = 30 mg MS (50 to 100 mg every 4-6 hours, not to exceed 400 mg/day)	Only in the oral form Side effects: see morphine May be habit forming

*Brand name
"Parenteral means intravenous (IV), intramuscular (IM), or subcutaneous (SC) injection.

TABLE II.3. Treatments for Side Effects of Narcotic Pain Relievers

Side Effect	Treatment	Preparation and Dose	Comments and Precautions
Nausea	Meclizine (Antivert*)/OTC**	Tablet: 12.5 or 25 mg Chewable tablet: 25 mg	Should not use in older adults, or persons with bladder obstruction or prostate problems,

Side Effect	Treatment	Preparation and Dose	Comments and Precautions
	(most effective when used to prevent nausea)	Dose: 12.5 mg every 8 hours to 25 mg every 6 hours	glaucoma, contact lenses, gastrointestinal tract obstruction, asthma, and other medical conditions. May cause drowsiness, worsen constipation, lower seizure threshold.
	Dimenhydrinate (Dramamine*)/OTC	Tablet: 50 mg	SEs same as meclizine
	(most effective when used to prevent nausea)	Dose: 50-150 mg every 4-6 hours as needed (do not exceed 400 mg total in 24 hours)	
	Scopolamine (Transderm Scop*)/OTC	1.5 mg/disc	SEs similar to meclizine
	(most effective when used to prevent nausea)	Apply disc to skin behind ear; change patch every three days; replace behind opposite ear	If nausea can be anticipated, place patch on 4 hours beforehand.
	Promethazine (Phenergan*)	Tablet or suppository: 12.5, 25, and 50 mg	SEs similar to meclizine
		Dose: 12.5- 25 mg every 4 to 6 hours	Lowers pain threshold and increases need for analgesia.
	Prochlorperazine (Compazine*)	Tablet: 5, 10, and 25 mg Suppository: 2.5, 5, and 25 mg	SEs similar to meclizine
			Has more SEs than promethazine, including dystonia and sedation.
		Dose: 5-10 mg every	
		6 to 8 hours (tablets); 12.5-25 mg every 4	

Side Effect	Treatment	Preparation and Dose	Comments and Precautions
	Ondansetron (Zofran*)	to 6 hours (suppository) Tablets: 4 and 8 mg Syrup: 4 mg/5 cc's Parenteral: 2 mg/cc Dose: 4 to 8 mg three times per day; 8 mg every 24 hours for extended use If nausea can be anticipated, take 30 min beforehand	Has fewer side effects than other drugs, but should not be used (or used with great caution) if liver disease, gastrointestinal problems, obese, pregnant, nursing, and if other medical conditions present.
	Alternative Treatments Ginger root/OTC (most effective when used to prevent nausea, rather than treat it) Acupressure	2 to 4 grams/day of fresh or dried root May take 0.5 to 1.0 gram prior to anticipated nausea There is a pressure point located on the inner forearm that may reduce nausea if pressed by fingers or a device that you can wear (Sea Bands* or Travel Aides*)	May increase bleeding, interfere with diabetes control, worsen gallbladder disease, and have other SEs. Pressure point is located on the inside of the forearm, about two thumb-widths above the wrist crease.
Excessive Sedation	Switch to another type of pain medication, or pain medication combination		
Itching (pruitis)	Diphenhydramine (Benadryl*)	Tablet: 25 and 50 mg Syrup: 12.5 mg/5 cc's Dose: 25-50 mg every 4 to 6 hours	SEs same as for meclizine; sedation makes bedtime use preferable. Avoid use in older adults.

Side Effect	Treatment	Preparation and Dose	Comments and Precautions
	Hydroxyzine (Vistaril*, Atarax*)	Tablet: 10, 25, 50, and 100 mg Capsule: 25, 50, and 100 mg	SEs same as for meclizine; sedation makes bedtime use preferable.
		Dose: 25-50 mg every 4-6 hours	Avoid use in older adults.
Constipation	Docusate sodium (Colace*)	Capsule: 50 and 100 mg Liquid: 150 mg/15 cc's Syrup: 50 mg/15 cc's	Especially useful for use with chronic opioid (narcotic) pain killers as a preventive measure
	Docusate sodium with Casanthranol (Pericolace*)	Dose: 100-200 mg twice daily Capsule: 100 mg docusate sodium with 30 mg casanthranol	Use for acute constipation (e.g., constipation already a problem) rather than plain docusate sodium.
		Syrup: 60 mg docusate sodium with 30 mg casanthranol/15 cc's (in 10 percent alcohol)	
		Dose: 1-2 capsules every 6 to 12 hours, or only at bedtime	
	Biscodyl (Dulcolax*) (if no relief after 72 hours despite other efforts)	Tablet: 5 mg Suppository: 5 and 10 mg	Do not crush or chew (since tablet is enteric coated).
	Sodium phosphate biphosphate (Fleets Phosphasoda*)	Dose: 5-15 mg tablet or suppository/day Enema: 135 cc's Solution: 30, 45, 90, 237 cc's	Avoid in people with low white blood cell counts. Dilute oral solution with equal amount of water.

Side Effect	Treatment	Preparation and Dose	Comments and Precautions
		Dose: 20-30 cc's orally; or 1 enema per rectum	Avoid enema in people with low white blood cell counts, or those with heart failure or fluid overload.
	Lactulose (Cephulac*, Duphalac*)	Syrup:10 gm/15 cc's	Avoid or extreme caution if gastrointestinal obstruction present.
	(last resort if no results and not impacted)	15-30 cc's from one to four times per day (maximum 60 cc/day)	
Respiratory Depression	Naloxone (Narcan*)	Parenteral (IV): 400 mcg/cc; may dilute 1:10 to ensure correct dosage	Ensure person is well-oxygenated.
		Dose 1-1.5 mcg/kg; May repeat in 3 min	May need to use as continuous infusion if long-acting opioid such as methadone.

*Brand name
**OTC = over-the-counter (nonprescription) medication

Notes

Chapter 1

1. <http://www.ampainsoc.org/whatsnew/conclude_road.htm>.
2. Bonica, J. J. (1987). In *Mastering Pain* (by Richard Sternbach). New York: Putnam, p. 11; Macek, C. (2001). The pain brigade. *DukeMed,* 1(1), 10.
3. Bonica, J. J. (1990). General considerations of chronic pain. *The Management of Pain.* Philadelphia: Lea and Febiger, pp. 180-208.
4. Lawrence, R. C., Hochberg, M. C., Kelsey, J .L., and McDuffie, F. C. (1987). Estimates of the prevalence of selected arthritic and musculoskeletal diseases in the United States. *Journal of Rheumatology,* 16, 427-441.
5. United Nations (1999). Population Aging 1999. UN Population Division, Department of Economic and Social Affairs, UN publication ST/ESA/SER.A/179, Sales No. 99. XIII.11, 99-93093, June.
6. Kroenke, K. and Price, R. K. (1993). Symptoms in the community. Prevalence, classification, and psychiatric comorbidity. *Archives of Internal Medicine,* 153, 2474-2480.
7. Kelly, J. and Raj, P. (1994). Chronic pain in a geriatric patient. *Pain Digest,* 4, 285-290.
8. Gureje, O., Von Korff, M., Simon, G.E., and Gater, R. (1998). Persistent pain and well-being: A World Health Organization Study in primary care. *Journal of the American Medical Association (JAMA),* 280(2):147-151.
9. Bove, G. and Nilsson, N. (1998). Spinal manipulation in the treatment of tension-type headache: A randomized controlled trial. *JAMA,* 280, 1576-1579; Shlay, J., Chaloner, K., Max, M. (1998). Acupuncture and amitriptyline for pain due to HIV-related peripheral neuropathy: A randomized controlled trial. *JAMA,* 280, 1590-1595.
10. Corran, T. M., Farrell, M. J., Helme, R., and Gibson, S. J. (1997). The classification of patients with chronic pain: Age as a contributing factor. *Clinical Journal of Pain,* 13, 207-214.
11. Bernabei, R., Gambassi, G., Lapane, K., Landi, F., Gatsonis, C., Dunlop, R., Lipsitz, L., Steel, K., and Mor, V. (1998). Management of pain in elderly patients with cancer. *JAMA,* 279, 1877-1882.
12. Hewitt, D. J. and Foley, K. M. (1997). Pain and pain management. In Cassel, C. K., Cohen, H. J., Larson, E. B., Meier, D. E., Resnick, N. M., Rubinstein, L. Z., and Sorensen, L.B. (Eds.), *Geriatric Medicine,* Third Edition. New York: Springer, p. 865-881.
13. Lamberg, L. (1998). New guidelines on managing chronic pain in older persons. *JAMA,* 280, 311-312.
14. Ferrell, B. A., Ferrell, B. R., and Osterweil, D. (1990). Pain in the nursing home. *Journal of the American Geriatrics Society,* 38, 409-414.

15. Fox, P. L., Parminder, R., and Jadad, A. R. (1999). Prevalence in treatment of pain in older adults in nursing homes and other long-term care institutions: A systematic review. *Canadian Medical Association Journal,* 160, 329-333.

16. Moss, M. S., Lawton, M. P., and Glicksman, A. (1991). The role of pain in the last year of life of older persons. *Journal of Gerontology,* 46, 51-57.

17. Foley, K. M. (1987). Pain syndromes in patients with cancer. *Medical Clinics of North America,* 71, 169-184.

18. See note 11.

19. Cooner, E. and Amorosi, S. (1997). *The Study of Pain in Older Americans.* New York: Louis Harris and Associates.

20. Portenoy, R. K. and Lesage, P. (1999). Management of cancer pain. *The Lancet,* 353, 1695-1700.

21. See note 9.

22. Shaughnessy, P. W. and Kramer, A. M. (1990). The increased needs of patients in nursing homes and patients receiving home health care. *New England Journal of Medicine,* 322, 21-27.

23. Locke, M. (2001). Suffering brings 1.5 M award: Jury agrees with family that California doctor under-medicated a dying lung cancer patient. *Associated Press,* June 15.

24. Merskey, H. (1979). Pain in terms: The list with definitions and a note on usage. Recommended by IASP Subcommittee on Taxonomy. *Pain,* 6, 249-252.

25. Jacobsen, L., Mariano, A. J., Chabal, C., and Chaney, E. F. (1997). Beyond the needle: Expanding the role of anesthesiologist in the management of chronic non-malignant pain. *Anesthesiology,* 87, 1210-1218.

26. Boden, S., Davis, D., Dina, T., Patronas, N., and Wiesel, S. (1990). Abnormal magnetic-resonance scans of the lumbar spine in asymptomatic subjects. A prospective investigation. *Journal of Bone and Joint Surgery,* 72, 403-408; Jensen, M., Brandt-Zawadski, M., Obuchowski, N., Modic, M., and Malakasian Ross, J. (1994). Magnetic resonance imaging of the lumbar spine in people with back pain. *New England Journal of Medicine,* 331, 69-73.

27. See note 23.

28. Roter, D. L., Hall, J. A., Kern, D. E., Barker, L. R., Cole, K. A., and Roca, R. P. (1995). Improving physicians' interviewing skills and reducing patients' emotional distress. *Archives of Internal Medicine,* 155, 1877-1884.

29. Turk, D. C. and Okifuji, A. (1999). Assessment of patients reporting of pain: An integrated perspective. *Lancet,* 353, 1784-1788.

30. Zborowski, M. (1952). Cultural components in responses to pain. *Journal of Social Issues,* 8, 16-30.

31. Kane, R. L., Ouslander, J. G., and Abrass, I. B. (1984). *Essentials of Clinical Geriatrics.* New York: McGraw-Hill Book Co.

32. Wolfe, F., Smythe, H. A., Yunus, M. B., Bennett, R. M., Bambardier, C., and Goldenberg, D. L. (1990). The American College of Rheumatology 1990 criteria for the classification of fibromyalgia. Report of the Multicenter Criteria Committee. *Arthritis and Rheumatism,* 33, 160-172.

33. Engel, C. C., von Korff, M., and Katon, W. J. (1996). Back pain and primary care: Predictors of high health care costs. *Pain,* 65, 197-204.

34. Weir, R., Brown, G., Tunks, E., Gafni, A., and Roberts, J. (1992). A profile of users of specialty pain clinic services: Predictors of use and cost estimates. *Journal of Clinical Epidemiology,* 45, 1399-1415.

35. Portenoy, R. K. and Lesage, P. (1999). Management of cancer pain. *Lancet,* 353, 1695-1700.

Chapter 8

1. Macek, C. (2001). The pain brigade. *DukeMed,* 1(1), 11.

2. Ibid., p. 15.

3. Turk, D. C. and Okifuji, A. (1999). Assessment of patients reporting of pain: An integrated perspective. *Lancet,* 353, 1784-1788.

4. Portenoy, R. K. and Lesage, P. (1999). Management of cancer pain. *Lancet,* 353, 1695-1700.

5. Melzack, R. (1987). The short-form McGill Pain Questionnaire. *Pain,* 30, 191-197.

6. Melzack, R. (1975). The McGill Pain Questionnaire: Major properties and scoring methods. *Pain,* 1, 277-299.

7. Turk, D. C. and Melzack, R. (1992). The measurement of pain in the assessment of people experiencing pain. In Turk D. C., and Melzack, R. (Eds.), *Handbook of Pain Assessment.* New York: Guilford Press.

8. Ferrell, B. A., Grant, M., and Dean, G. E. (1996). "Bone tired." The experience of fatigue and its impact on quality of life. *Oncology Nursing Forum,* 23, 1539-1547.

9. AGS Panel (1998). The management of chronic pain in older adults (by the American Geriatric Society panel on chronic pain in older persons). *Journal of the American Geriatric Society,* 46, 635-651.

10. Reuters Health report, February 22, 2000. Online: <http://www.brainland.com/indiv_news.cfm?ID=161>.

11. Li, P. and Zhuo, M. (1998). Silent glutamatergic synapses and nociception in mammalian spinal cord. *Nature,* 393 (6686), 695-698.

12. Reuters Health report, June 17, 1998.

Chapter 9

1. Ashburn, M. A. and Staats, P. S. (1999). Management of chronic pain. *The Lancet,* 353, 1865-1869.

2. AGS Panel (1998). The management of chronic pain in older adults. *Journal of the American Geriatric Society,* 46, 635-651.

3. Ibid.

4. Wolfe, M. M., Lichtenstein, D. R., and Singh, G. (1999). Gastrointestinal toxicity of nonsteroidal antiinflammatory drugs. *New England Journal of Medicine,* 340, 1888-1899.

5. Greenberger, N. J. (1997). Update in gastroenterology. *Annals of Internal Medicine,* 125, 827-834.

6. Schnitzer, T. J. (2001). Cyclooxygenase-2–specific inhibitors: Are they safe? *American Journal of Medicine,* 110(1A), 46S-49S.

7. Kivitz, A., Schnitzer, T., Greenwald, M. Fleischmann, R., Matzura-Wolfe, D., Polis, A., Dixon, M., Dobbins, T., and Geba, G. (2001). Rofecoxib provided superior relief of symptoms of osteoarthritis (OA) compared to celecoxib. *Journal of the American Geriatrics Society,* 49(4), S126.

8. Max, M. B. (1995). Thirteen consecutive well-designed randomized trials showing that antidepressants reduce pain in diabetic neuropathy and post-herpetic neuralgia. *Pain Forum,* 4, 248-253.

9. Onghena, P. and Van Houdenhove, B. (1992). Antidepressant-induced analgesia in chronic non-malignant pain: A meta-analysis of 39 placebo-controlled studies. *Pain,* 49(2), 205-219.

10. Fishbain, D. A., Cutler, R. B., Rosomoff, H. L., and Rosomoff, R. (1998). Do antidepressants have an analgesic effect in psychogenic pain and somatoform pain disorder? A meta-analysis. *Psychosomatic Medicine,* 60(4), 503-509.

11. See note 9.

12. Max, M. B. (1994). Antidepressants and analgesics. In Fields, H. L., and Liebeskind, J. C. (Eds.), *Pharmacological Approaches to the Treatment of Chronic Pain: New Concepts and Critical Issues: Progress in Pain Research and Management,* Volume 1. Seattle: International Association for the Study of Pain (IASP) Press, pp. 229-246.

13. Goldenberg, D., Mayskiy, M., Mossey, C. (1996). A randomized, double-blind crossover trial of fluoxetine and amitriptyline in the treatment of fibromyalgia. *Arthritis and Rheumatism,* 39, 1852-1859.

14. Goli, V. (2000). *Drug helps chronic pain due to diabetic neuropathy.* Presented at the 60th Scientific Session of the American Diabetes Association, San Antonio, TX, July 3.

15. Bates, B. (2001). Consider tricyclics, anticonvulsants to treat pain. *Clinical Psychiatry News,* 29(5), 33.

16. DeMott, K. (2001). Opioids still worthwhile despite street-drug taint. *Clinical Psychiatry News,* 29(6), 46.

17. Lynch, M. E. (2001). Antidepressants as analgesics: A review of randomized controlled trials. *Journal of Psychiatry and Neuroscience,* 26(1), 30-36.

18. Galer, B. S., Rowbotham, M., Perander, J., Devers, A., and Friedman, E. (2000). Topical diclofenac patch relieves minor sports injury pain: Results of a multicenter controlled clinical trial. *Journal of Pain and Symptom Management,* 19(4), 287-294.

19. Dellemijn, P., van Duijn, H., and Vanneste, J. (1998). Prolonged treatment with transdermal fentanyl in neuropathic pain. *Journal of Pain and Symptom Management,* 16, 220-229.

20. Popp, B. and Portenoy, R. K. (1996). Management of chronic pain in the elderly: Pharmacology of opioid and other analgesic drugs. In Ferrell, B. R. and Ferrell, B. A. (Eds.), *Pain in the Elderly.* Seattle: International Association for the Study of Pain (IASP) Press, pp. 21-34.

21. Joranson, D. and Gilson, A. M. (1997). State intractable pain policy: Current status. *American Pain Society Bulletin,* 7, 7-9.

22. Federation of State Medical Boards of the U.S. (1998). Model guidelines for the use of controlled substances for the treatment of pain. Euless, TX: Federation of State Medical Boards of the United States, Inc. <http://www.fsmb.org/new.htm>.

23. Macek, C. (2001). The pain brigade. *DukeMed,* 1(1), 10.

24. Edell, D. (2000). Improvements in treating chronic pain. *Health Central,* July 18, 2000 <http://www.healthcentral.com/drdean/deanfulltexttopics.cfm?id= 38001>.

25. AAPM (1997). American Academy of Pain Medicine and American Pain Society (APS). The use of opioids for the treatment of chronic pain. Glenview, IL: AAPM and APS (see also *Clinical Journal of Pain,* 13, 6-8).

26. McQuay, H. (1999). Opioids in pain management. *Lancet,* 353, 2229-2232.

27. Lamberg, L. (1998). New guidelines on managing chronic pain in older persons. *Journal of the American Medical Association,* 280, 311-312.

28. See note 26.

29. Ibid.

30. Moulin, D. E., Iezzi, A., Amireh, R., Sharpe, W. K., Boyd, D., and Merskey, H. (1996). Randomized trial of oral morphine for chronic non-cancer pain. *Lancet,* 347, 143-147.

31. See note 26.

32. Eisenach, J. C., DuPen, S., Dubois, M., Miguel, R., and Allin, D. (1995). Epidural clonidine analgesia for intractable cancer pain. The epidural clonidine study group. *Pain,* 61, 391-399.

33. Schnitzer, T. J., Kamin, M., and Olson, W. H. (1999). Tramadol allows reduction of naproxen dose among patients with naproxen-responsive osteoarthritis pain: A randomized, double-blind, placebo-controlled study. *Arthritis and Rheumatism,* 42, 1370-1377.

34. Arnst, C. (1999). Conquering pain: New discoveries and treatments offer hope. *Business Week,* March 1, pp. 102-110.

35. See note 2.

36. See note 34.

37. Ibid.

38. Lipsky, P., van der Heijde, D., St. Clair, W., et al. (2000). 102-wk clinical and radiologic results from the ATTRACT trial: A 2-year randomized, controlled, phase 3 trial of infliximab (Remicade) in patients with active RA despite MTX. Program and abstracts from the 64th Annual Scientific Meeting of the American College of Rheumatology (Oct. 29-Nov. 2, Philadelphia, Pennsylvania, Abstract 1216).

39. Genovese, M., Martin, R., and Fleischmann, R., et al. (2000). Embrel (etanercept) vs. methotrexate (MTX) in early rheumatoid arthritis (ERA trial): Two-year follow-up. Program and abstracts from the 64th Annual Scientific Meeting of the American College of Rheumatology (Oct. 29-Nov. 2, Philadelphia, Pennsylvania, Abstract 1217).

Chapter 10

1. Fishbain, D., Cutler, R., Rosomoff, H. L., and Rosomoff, R. S. (1997). Chronic pain-associated depression: Antecedent or consequence of chronic pain? A review. *Clinical Journal of Pain,* 13, 116-137.

2. Ibid.

3. Romano, J. M. and Turner, J. A. (1985). Chronic pain and depression: Does the evidence support a relationship? *Psychological Bulletin,* 97, 18-34.

4. Chapman, C. R. and Gavrin, J. (1999). Suffering: The contributions of persistent pain. *Lancet,* 353, 2233-2237.

5. Ibid.

6. See note 3.

7. Morin, C. M. (1993). *Insomnia: Psychological Assessment and Management*. New York: Guilford Press.

8. Atkinson, J. H., Ancoli-Israel, S., and Slater, M. (1988). Subjective sleep disturbance in chronic pain. *Clinical Journal of Pain, 4*, 225-232.

9. Morin, C. M., Gibson, D., and Wade, J. (1998). Self-reported sleep and mood disturbance in chronic pain patients. *Clinical Journal of Pain, 14*, 311-314.

10. Morin, C. M., Kowatch, R. A., and Wade, J. (1989). Behavioral management of sleep disturbances secondary to chronic pain. *Journal of Behavioral Therapy and Experimental Psychology, 20*, 295-302.

11. Coughlin, A. M., Badura, A. S., Fleischer, T. D., and Guck, T. P. (2000). Multidisciplinary treatment of chronic pain patients: Its efficacy in changing patient locus of control. *Archives of Physical Medicine and Rehabilitation*, 81(6):739-740.

12. Krause, N., Herzog, A. R., and Baker, E. (1992). Providing support to others and well-being in later life. *Journal of Gerontology, 47*, 300-311.

13. Koenig, H. G., Pargament, K. I., and Nielsen, J. (1998). Religious coping and health status in medically ill hospitalized older adults. *Journal of Nervous and Mental Disease, 186*, 513-521.

14. Leibing, E., Pfingsten, M., Bartman, U., Rueger, U., and Schuessler, G. (1999). Cognitive-behavioral treatment in selected rheumatoid arthritis outpatients. *Clinical Journal of Pain, 15*, 58-66.

15. Mullen, P. D., Laville, E. A., and Biddle, A. K. (1987). Efficacy of psychoeducational interventions on pain depression and disability in people with arthritis. A meta-analysis. *Journal of Rheumatology, 14* (supplement 15), 33-39.

16. Arnstein, P., et al. (2000). Cognitive behavioral treatment for chronic pain (reported by Guang-Shing Cheng). *Clinical Psychiatry News, 28*(2), 23.

17. Backus, W. and Chapin, M. (2000). *Telling Yourself the Truth*. Minneapolis, MN: Bethany House.

18. Bradley, L. A., Young, L. D., Anderson, K. O., Turner, R. A., Agudelo, C. A., McDaniel, L. K., Pisko, E. J., Semble, E. L., and Morgan, T. M. (1987). Effects of psychological therapy on pain behavior of rheumatoid arthritis patients. Treatment outcome and six-month follow-up. *Arthritis and Rheumatism, 30*, 1105-1114.

19. Jamison, R. N. and Virts, K. L. (1990). The influence of family support on chronic pain. *Behavior Research and Therapy, 28*, 283-287.

20. Rene, J., Weinberger, M., Mazzuca, S. A., Brandt, K. D., and Katz, B. P. (1992). Reduction of joint pain in patients with osteoarthritis who have received monthly telephone calls from late personnel and whose medical treatment regimens have remained stable. *Arthritis and Rheumatism, 35*, 511-515; Weinberger, M., Tierney, W. M., Cowper, P. A., Katz, D. P., and Booher, P. A. (1993). Cost-effectiveness of increased telephone contact for patients with loss to arthritis: A randomized, controlled trial. *Arthritis and Rheumatism, 26*, 243-246.

21. Melzack, R. (1982). Recent concepts of pain. *Journal of Medicine, 13*, 147-160.

22. Bradley, L. A., Young, L. D., Anderson, K. O., McDaniel, L. K., Turner, R. A., Agudelo, C. A. (1984). Psychological approaches to the management of arthritis pain. *Social Science and Medicine, 19*, 1353-1360.

23. Keefe, F. J. and Williams, D. A. (1990). A comparison of coping strategies in chronic pain patients in different age groups. *Journal of Gerontology, 45*, 161-165.

24. Cook, A. J. (1998). Cognitive-behavioral pain management for elderly nursing home residents. *Journal of Gerontology,* 53, P51-P59.

25. Benson, H. (1975). *The Relaxation Response.* NY: William Morrow.

26. Cogan, R., Cogan, D., Waltz, W., and McCue, M. (1987). Effects of laughter and relaxation on discomfort thresholds. *Journal of Behavioral Medicine,* 10, 139-144.

27. Berk, L. S., Tan, S. A., Fry, W. F., Napier, B. J., Lee, J. W., Hubbard, R. W., Lewis, J. E., and Eby, W. C. (1989). Neuroendocrine and stress hormone changes during mirthful laughter. *American Journal of the Medical Sciences,* 298, 390-396.

Chapter 11

1. Eisenberg, D. M., Davis, R. B., Ettner, S. L., Appel, S., Wilkey, S., Rompay, M. V., and Kessler, R. C. (1998). Trends in alternative medicine use in the United States, 1990-1997. *JAMA,* 280, 1569-1575.

2. Ibid.

3. Referenced in a presentation given by Dr. James W. Jefferson, Distinguished Senior Scientist, Madison Institute of Medicine, for *Audio-Digest Psychiatry,* 30(1), p. 2 of transcript.

4. Ibid.

5. Pittler, M. H. and Ernst, E. (2000). Efficacy of kava extract for treating anxiety: Systematic review and meta-analysis. *Journal of Clinical Psychopharmacology,* 20(1), 84-89.

6. Graedon, J., Graedon, T. (2001). *The People's Pharmacy.* New York: St. Martin's Press, pp. 38-40.

7. Imperio, W. A. (2001). St. John's wort varies by brand. *Clinical Psychiatry News,* 29(5), 51.

8. Imperio, W. A. (2001). St. John's wort fails first placebo trial. *Clinical Psychiatry News,* 29(5), 1-2.

9. Hypericum Depression Trial Study Group (2002). Effect of *Hypericum perforatum* (St. John's wort) in Major Depressive Disorder: A randomized controlled trial. *Journal of the American Medical Association,* 287(14): 1807-1814.

10. Brzeski, M., Madhok, R., and Capell, H. A. Evening primrose oil in patients with rheumatoid arthritis and side-effects of non-steroidal anti-inflammatory drugs. *British Journal of Rheumatology,* 1991; 30(5): 370-2; Ariza-Ariza, R., Mestanza-Peralta, M., and Cardiol, M. H. Omega-3 fatty acids in rheumatoid arthritis: An overview. *Seminars in Arthritis and Rheumatism,* 1998; 27:366-70.

11. Stoll, A. *The Omega-3 Connection.* New York: Simon and Schuster, 2001, pp. 226-252.

12. McAlindon, T. E., LaValley, M. P., Gulin, J. P., and Felson, D. T. (2000). Glucosamine and chondroitin for treatment of osteoarthritis: A systematic quality assessment and meta-analysis. *JAMA,* 283(11):1469-1475.

13. Reginster, J.-Y., Deroisy, R., Paul, I., Lee, R. L., Henroitoin, Y., Giacovelli G., et al. (1999). Glucosamine sulfate significantly reduces progression of knee osteoarthritis over 3 years: A large, randomised, placebo-controlled, prospective trial. *Arthritis and Rheumatism,* 42:S400.

14. NIH awards study on glucosamine/chondroitin sulfate for knee osteoarthritis [press release]. Bethesda, MD: National Institutes of Health; September 15, 1999.

15. AGS Panel 1998.

16. Loitman, J. E. (2000). Pain management: Beyond pharmacology to acupuncture and hypnosis. *JAMA, 283*, 118-119.

17. ter Riet, G., Kleijnen, J., Knipschild, P. (1990). Acupuncture and chronic pain: A criteria-based meta-analysis. *Journal of Clinical Epidemiology, 43*(11), 1191-1199.

18. van Tulder, M. W., Cherkin, D. C., Berman, B., Lao, L., and Koes, B. W. (1999). The effectiveness of acupuncture in the management of acute and chronic low back pain: A systematic review within the framework of the Cochrane Collaboration Back Review Group. *Spine,* 24(11), 1113-1123.

19. Ramnarine-Singh, S. (1999). The surgical significance of therapeutic touch. *Association of Perioperative Registered Nurses (AORN) Journal,* 69(2):358-369.

20. See note 16.

21. Rosa, L., Rosa, E., Sarner, L., and Barrett, S. (1998). A close look at therapeutic touch. *JAMA,* 279(13):1005-1010.

22. Brown, C. (2000). Magnets and chronic pelvic pain. Presented at the annual meeting of the American College of Obstetrics and Gynecology, San Francisco, May 22.

23. Collacott, E. A., Zimmerman, J. T., White, D. W., and Rindone, J. P. (2000). Bipolar permanent magnets for the treatment of chronic low back pain: A pilot study. *JAMA,* 283(10):1322-1325.

24. Andersson, G. B., Lucente, T., Davis, A. M., Kappler, R. E., Lipton, J. A., and Leurgans, S. (1999). A comparison of osteopathic spinal manipulation with standard care for patients with low back pain. *New England Journal of Medicine,* 341(19):1426-1431.

25. Bove, G. and Nilsson, N. (1998). Spinal manipulation in the treatment of episodic tension-type headache: A randomized controlled trial. *JAMA,* 280(18):1576-1579.

Chapter 12

1. Krames, E. S. (1999). Interventional pain management. Appropriate when less invasive therapies fail to provide adequate analgesia. *Medical Clinics of North America* 1999, 83, 787-808.

2. Jacobsen, L., Mariano, A. J., Chabal, C., and Chaney, E. F. (1997). Beyond the needle: Expanding the role of anesthesiologist in the management of chronic non-malignant pain. *Anesthesiology,* 87, 1210-1218.

3. Macek, C. (2001). The pain brigade. *DukeMed,* 1(1), 13.

4. Barolat, G., and Sharan, A. D. (2000). Future trends in spinal cord stimulation. *Neurological Research,* 22:279-284.

5. Tseng, S. H. (2000). Treatment of chronic pain by spinal cord stimulation. *Journal of the Formosan Medical Association,* 99: 267-271.

6. Fanciullo, G. J., Rose, R. J., Lunt, P. G., Whalen, P. K., and Ross, E. (1999). The state of implantable pain therapies in the United States: A nationwide survey of academic teaching programs. *Anesthesia and Analgesia,* 88, 1311-1316.

7. Saitoh, Y., Shibata, M., and Hirano, S. (2000). Motor cortex stimulation for central and peripheral deafferentation. *Journal of Neurosurgery* 2000, 92,15155.

8. Garcia-Larrea, L., Peryon, R., and Mertens, P. (1999). Electrical stimulation of motor cortex for pain control: A combined PET-scan an electrophysiological study. *Pain,* 83, 259-273.

9. Nguyen, J. P., Lefaucheur, J. P., Decq, P., and Uchiyama, T. (1999). Chronic motor cortex stimulation in the treatment of central and neuropathic pain. Correlations between clinical, electrophysiological and anatomical data. *Pain,* 82, 245-251.

10. Finegold, A. A., Mannes, A. J., and Iadarola, M. J. (1999). A paracrine paradigm for in vivo gene therapy in the central nervous system: Treatment of chronic pain. *Human Gene Therapy,* 10(7):1251-1257.

11. Arnst, C. (1999). Conquering pain: New discoveries and treatments that offer hope. *Business Weekly,* March 1, p. 103.

Chapter 13

1. Lane, N. E. and Thompson, J. M. (1997). Management of osteoarthritis in the primary-care setting: An evidence-based approach to treatment. *American Journal of Medicine,* 103(6A Supplement), 25S-30S.

2. Andersen, S. J. and Cannon, G. W. (2001). Efficacy and tolerability of cyclooxygenase-2 inhibitors in the treatment of osteoarthritis in the elderly. *Clinical Geriatrics,* 9, 20-36.

3. Gonzalez, G. R. and Portenoy, R. K. (1993). Selection of analgesics therapies in rheumatoid arthritis: The role of opioid medications. *Arthritis Care and Research,* 6, 223-238.

4. Foley, K. M. (1991). Clinical tolerance to opioids. In Basbaum, A. I., Besson, J. M. (Eds.), *Towards a New Pharmacotherapy of Pain.* New York: John Wiley and Sons, pp. 181-203.

5. Ytterberg, S. R., Mahowald, M. L., and Woods, S. R. (1998). Codeine and oxycodone use in patients with chronic rheumatic disease pain. *Arthritis and Rheumatism,* 41, 1603-1612.

6. Ibid.

7. Ibid.

8. Ibid.

9. Turk, D. C., Brody, M. C., and Okifuji, E. A. (1994). Physicians' attitudes and practices regarding the long-term prescribing of opioids for non-cancer pain. *Pain,* 59, 201-208.

10. Portenoy, R. K. (1990). Chronic opioid therapy in non-malignant pain. *Journal of Pain and Symptom Management,* 5 Suppl: S46-S62.

11. Weinberger, M., Tierney, W. M., Cowper, P. A., Katz, D. P., and Booher, P. A. (1993). Cost-effectiveness of increased telephone contact for patients with loss to arthritis: A randomized, controlled trial. *Arthritis and Rheumatism,* 26, 243-246.

12. Millea, P. J. and Holloway, R. L. (2000). Treating fibromyalgia. *American Family Physician,* 62, 1575-1582, 1587.

13. Ibid.

14. Berman, B. M., Ezzo, J., Hadhazy, V., and Swyer, J. P. (1999). Is acupuncture effective in the treatment of fibromyalgia? *Journal of Family Practice,* 48, 213-218.

15. Linton-Dahlof, P., Linde, M., and Dahlof, C. (2000). Withdrawal therapy improves chronic daily headache associated with long-term use of headache medication: A retrospective study. *Cephalalgia,* 20(7), 658-662.

16. Ward, T. M. (2000). Providing relief from headache. *Postgraduate Medicine,* 108(3), 121-128; Headache Classification Committee of the International Headache Society (1988). Classification and diagnostic criteria for headache disorders, cranial neuralgias and facial pain. *Cephalalgia,* 8 (Suppl. 7), 1-96.

17. Portenoy, R. K. and Lesage, P. (1999). Management of cancer pain. *Lancet,* 353, 1695-1700.

18. Cleeland, C. S. (1998). Undertreatment of cancer pain in elderly patients. *JAMA,* 279, 1914-1915.

19. Sykes, J., Johnson, R., and Hanks, G. W. (1997). ABC's of palliative care: Difficult pain problems. *British Medical Journal,* 315, 867-869.

20. Portenoy, R. K., Dole, V., Joseph, H., Lowinson, J., Rice, C., Siegel, S., and Richman, B. L. (1997). Pain management and chemical dependency: Evolving perspectives. *JAMA,* 278, 592-593.

21. WHO (1996). World Health Organization's *Cancer Pain Relief,* Second Edition. Geneva: World Health Organization.

22. Foley, K. M. and Portenoy, R. K. (1993) World Health Organization—International Association for the Study of Pain: Joint initiatives in cancer pain relief. *Journal of Pain and Symptom Management,* 8(6), 335-339.

23. Jadad, M. R. and Browman, G. P. (1995). The WHO analgesic ladder for cancer pain management. *JAMA,* 274, 870-873.

24. See note 18.

25. Kaiko, R. F. (1980). Age and morphine analgesia skin cancer patients with post-operative pain. *Clinical Pharmacology and Therapy,* 28, 823-826; see also Ventafridda, V., Saita, L., Barletta, L., Sbanotto, A., DeConno, F. (1989). Clinical observations on controlled release morphine in cancer pain. *Journal of Pain and Symptom Management,* 4, 124-129.

26. Kalso, E., Heisknen, T., Rantio, M., Rosenberg, P. H, and Vainio, A. (1996). Epidural and subcutaneous morphine in the management of cancer pain: A double-blind cross-over study. *Pain,* 67, 443-449.

27. Hanks, G. W. (1987). Opioid analgesics in the management of pain in patients with cancer: A review. *Palliative Medicine,* 1, 1-25.

28. Vanegas, G., Ripamonti, C., Sbanotto, A., and DeConno, F. (1998). Side effects of morphine administration in cancer patients. *Cancer Nursing,* 21, 289-297.

29. Vainio, A. and Auvinen, A., with members of the Symptom Prevalence Group (1996). Prevalence of symptoms among patients with advanced cancer: An international collaborative group. *Journal of Pain and Symptom Management,* 12, 3-10.

30. DeMott, K. (2001). Opioids still worthwhile despite street-drug taint. *Clinical Psychiatry News,* 29(6), 46.

Chapter 14

1. Peterson, E. H. (1994). *The Message: The New Testament in Contemporary Language.* Colorado Springs, CO: NavPress Publishing Group, p. 353.

2. DC Talk (1999). *Jesus Freaks: Stories of Those Who Stood for Jesus: The Ultimate Jesus Freaks.* Minneapolis, MN: Bethany House Publishers.

3. Author unknown. Circulated on the Internet.

4. Schaefer, E. (1978). *Affliction.* Old Tappan, NJ: Fleming H. Revell Company.

5. Uchino, B. N., Cacioppo, J. R., and Kiecolt-Glaser, J. K. (1996). The relationship between social support and physiological processes: A review with emphasis on underlying mechanisms and implications for health. *Psychological Bulletin,* 119, 488-531; Sapolsky, R. M., Alberts, S. C., and Altman, J. (1997). Hypercortisolism associated with social subordinance or social isolation among wild baboons. *Archives of General Psychiatry,* 54, 1137-1143; Kiecolt-Glaser, J. K., Ricker, D., and George, J. (1984). Urinary cortisol levels, cellular immunocompetence, and loneliness in psychiatric inpatients. *Psychosomatic Medicine,* 46, 15-23.

6. Ibid.

7. Benson, H. and Stark, M. (1997). *Timeless Healing: The Power and Biology of Belief.* New York: Simon and Schuster.

8. Kabat-Zinn, J., Lipworth, L., and Burney, R. (1985). The clinical use of mindfulness meditation for the self-regulation of chronic pain. *Journal of Behavioral Medicine,* 8, 163-190.

9. Stephan, B. D. (2001). *Meditation for Christians.* Riverdale, NE: Watchfulness Publishing.

Chapter 15

1. Ashburn, M. A. and Staats, P. S. (1999). Management of chronic pain. *Lancet,* 353, 1865-1869.

2. DC Talk (1999). *Jesus Freaks: Stories of Those Who Stood for Jesus: The Ultimate Jesus Freaks.* Minneapolis, MN: Bethany House Publishers.

3. Bunyan, J. (1994 edition). *The Pilgrim's Progress.* Old Tappen, NJ: Fleming H. Revel Company.

4. Winter, D. (1971). *Closer than a Brother* (reinterpretation of the devotional classic, *Practicing the Presence of God* by Brother Lawrence). Wheaton, IL: Harold Shaw Publishers.

5. Kempis, T. (1998 translation by Joseph Tylenda). *The Imitation of Christ.* New York: Random House.

6. Vicente, Peter J. (Ed.). *American Pain Society Bulletin.* Glenview, IL: American Pain Society. (This is a bimonthly publication.)

7. Lande, S. D. and Kulich, R. J. (Eds.) (2000). *Managed Care and Pain.* Glenview, IL: American Pain Society.

8. Benjamin, L. J., Dampier, C. D., Jacox, A., Odesina, V., Phoenix, D., Shapiro, B. S., Stafford, M., and Treadwell, M. (n.d.). *Guidelines for the Management of Acute and Chronic Pain in Sickle-Cell Disease.* Glenview, IL: American Pain Society.

9. American Pain Society (2002). *Principles of Analgesic Use in the Treatment of Acute Pain and Cancer Pain,* Fourth Edition. Glenview, IL: American Pain Society.

Appendix I

1. *The New International Version.* Grand Rapids, MI: Zondervan Publishing House, 1984.

2. *The King James Version.* Cambridge: Cambridge, 1769.

Index

Page numbers followed by the letter "t" indicate tables.

Spinal endoscopy, 190-191
Spinal fusion, 190
Spinal injury, pain, 1-2
Spinal roots, neurosurgery, 188
Spinal stenosis, back pain, 24
Spinal surgeries, types of, 189-191
Spiritual rituals, spiritual strategies, 260-261
Spiritual strategies
    and chronic pain, 2, 3, 154, 227, 260-262
    components of, 228-234
Spiritual visualization, spiritual strategies, 261
Spondylosis, back pain, 24
St. John's Wort, herbal remedy, 69-170
Stadol NS
    for cluster headaches, 217
    for migraine treatment, 215
Stress
    and chronic pain, 148
    psychogenic pain, 17
Submission, spiritual component, 228-229
"Substance P," 141
Suffering
    description of, 146-148
    and pain, 1
    spiritual activities, 234
Suicidal ideation
    chronic pain, 146
    cluster headaches,
Sumatriptan (Imitrex)
    for cluster headaches, 217
    for migraines, 214, 215
Suppositories, for migraines, 215
Surgery
    Bob's story, 40, 43
    Jackie's story, 87, 90, 91, 93
    Joan's story, 103, 104, 105
    negative consequences of, 192
    osteoarthritis treatment, 206
    pain control, 191
    pain management, 251, 258-259
Surgical procedures, and chronic pain, 2, 3, 185-191
Sweating, morphine side effect, 221-222
Sympathectomy, neurosurgery, 187

Tegretol
    as adjuvant drug, 223
    anticonvulsant, 132, 281t-282t
Telling Yourself the Truth, 153
Tendinitis, 6-7, 20
Tension headaches
    pain syndrome, 22
    treatment of, 216
Therapeutic touch (TT), 3, 180-181
1 Thessalonians, on suffering, 269
2 Timothy, on suffering, 269
Tissue damage, 14, 19
Tolectin, NSAID, 128
Tolerance, narcotic analgesics, 203, 205
Tolmetin (Tolectin), NSAID, 128
Topical treatments
    for chronic pain, 133, 283t
    for osteoarthritis, 203
Tramadol (Ultram)
    chronic pain, 139, 288t
    for osteoarthritis treatment, 204
    for WHO protocol, 219
Transcutaneous nerve stimulator (TENS)
    Bob's story, 42, 192
    chronic back pain, 218
    chronic pain, 126, 253
    description of, 192-193
    Joan's story, 107, 192
    osteoarthritis treatment, 205
    pain treatment, 143
Treatment
    medications, 123-142, 279t-292t
    pain assessment, 117-118
    psychological, 151-158
Triamcinolone hexacetonide, osteoarthritis injections, 203
Tricyclic antidepressants
    for chronic pain, 130, 133
    for headaches, 211
    for osteoarthritis, 202-203
Trigeminal neuralgia, surgery, 185
Tumor necrosis factor (TNF), 142
Tylenol
    acute pain, 124
    chronic pain, 126-127, 133, 252, 279t
    for headaches, 211
    for osteoporosis, 201-202

CHRONIC PAIN
Biomedical and Spiritual Approaches

_____in hardbound at $37.46 (regularly $49.95) (ISBN: 0-7890-1638-9)

_____in softbound at $18.71 (regularly $24.95) (ISBN: 0-7890-1639-7)

Or order online and use Code HEC25 in the shopping cart.

COST OF BOOKS_____

OUTSIDE USA/CANADA/ MEXICO: ADD 20%_____

POSTAGE & HANDLING_____
(US: $4.00 for first book & $1.50 for each additional book)
Outside US: $5.00 for first book & $2.00 for each additional book)

SUBTOTAL_____

in Canada: add 7% GST_____

STATE TAX_____
(NY, OH & MIN residents, please add appropriate local sales tax)

FINAL TOTAL_____
(If paying in Canadian funds, convert using the current exchange rate, UNESCO coupons welcome.)

☐ **BILL ME LATER:** ($5 service charge will be added)
(Bill-me option is good on US/Canada/Mexico orders only; not good to jobbers, wholesalers, or subscription agencies.)

☐ Check here if billing address is different from shipping address and attach purchase order and billing address information.

Signature_____

☐ **PAYMENT ENCLOSED: $**_____

☐ **PLEASE CHARGE TO MY CREDIT CARD.**

☐ Visa ☐ MasterCard ☐ AmEx ☐ Discover
☐ Diner's Club ☐ Eurocard ☐ JCB

Account # _____

Exp. Date_____

Signature_____

Prices in US dollars and subject to change without notice.

NAME_____

INSTITUTION_____

ADDRESS_____

CITY_____

STATE/ZIP_____

COUNTRY_____ COUNTY (NY residents only)_____

TEL_____ FAX_____

E-MAIL_____

May we use your e-mail address for confirmations and other types of information? ☐ Yes ☐ No
We appreciate receiving your e-mail address and fax number. Haworth would like to e-mail or fax special discount offers to you, as a preferred customer. **We will never share, rent, or exchange your e-mail address or fax number.** We regard such actions as an invasion of your privacy.

Order From Your Local Bookstore or Directly From
The Haworth Press, Inc.
10 Alice Street, Binghamton, New York 13904-1580 • USA
TELEPHONE: 1-800-HAWORTH (1-800-429-6784) / Outside US/Canada: (607) 722-5857
FAX: 1-800-895-0582 / Outside US/Canada: (607) 722-6362
E-mailto: getinfo@haworthpressinc.com
PLEASE PHOTOCOPY THIS FORM FOR YOUR PERSONAL USE.
http://www.HaworthPress.com   BOF02